NHA PHLEBOTOMY EXAM PREP:

PAGE 2 INTRODUCTION:

PAGE 5 Section 1: Safety and Compliance:

PAGE 17 Section 2: Patient Preparation:

PAGE 26 Section 3: Routine Blood Collections:

PAGE 34 Section 4: Special Collections and Point of Care Testing:

PAGE 46 Section 5: Processing and Handling:

PAGE 58 Exam Prep Section:

INTRODUCTION:

Welcome to your journey towards acing the NHA Certified Phlebotomy Technician (CPT) Examination. You hold in your hands a tool that's been meticulously designed to light the path ahead, clarify your doubts, and arm you with the knowledge needed to conquer this challenge.

In the pages to come, we'll delve deep into the realms of safety and compliance, patient preparation, routine blood collections, special collections, point-of-care testing, and the processing and handling of samples. We aim to cover every nook and cranny of the exam content, turning the intimidating into the familiar.

We understand that the journey may seem daunting. There might be times when you question your capacity to succeed. But remember, success isn't the absence of failure—it's the resilience to keep going despite it. In this guide, not only will we equip you with the technical knowledge required, but we will also provide tips on how to handle setbacks, build resilience, and stay on course towards your goal.

As we unravel the complexities of each topic, we'll illustrate with real-world examples, bringing theoretical concepts to life. You'll find the subject matter to be more relatable and easier to remember.

Remember, the pursuit of your dreams is a journey filled with opportunities for learning and growth. This guide is a significant step in that journey. As you flip through these pages and soak in the knowledge, envision the success that awaits you on the other side. Your dreams are valid, and your goal of becoming a Certified Phlebotomy Technician is entirely within your reach.

The path to success isn't always smooth or straightforward—it might indeed involve throwing a few metaphorical rocks at obstacles that stand in your way. But with persistence, dedication, and the right resources, those obstacles can be overcome.

We're with you every step of the way, and we believe in your potential to master the content and succeed in the exam. Let's embark on this journey together, turning challenges into triumphs, and dreams into reality.

The purpose of this study guide is manifold. First and foremost, it serves as a comprehensive tool to prepare you for the NHA Certified Phlebotomy Technician (CPT) Examination. This guide will provide you with the knowledge and understanding necessary to navigate the exam confidently and effectively.

The guide aims to demystify each topic covered in the exam, breaking them down into digestible sections. It serves to clarify complex concepts, present real-world scenarios, and reinforce critical points - making the learning process more engaging and less daunting.

Additionally, this guide offers study strategies and test-taking tips to help optimize your exam performance. It's not just about knowing the material, but understanding how to apply your knowledge effectively in an exam setting.

Lastly, this guide acts as a supplement to your existing coursework and practical training. It's designed to bridge any gaps, reinforce what you've already learned, and provide additional insights.

In essence, this study guide is your trusty companion on your journey towards becoming a Certified Phlebotomy Technician, helping you navigate the path to success in the exam.

Here's to your success—let's get started!

The National Healthcareer Association's (NHA) Certified Phlebotomy Technician (CPT) Examination is a rigorous and comprehensive assessment for individuals aspiring to work as Phlebotomy Technicians. Here's an in-depth look at what the exam covers:

1. Safety and Compliance (15% of the exam)

In this section, you'll be assessed on your knowledge of safety protocols and legal guidelines related to phlebotomy. Topics include:

- Infection control: Understanding of how to prevent infection transmission, including hand hygiene, use of personal protective equipment (PPE), and safe disposal of sharps and biohazard waste.
- Safety regulations: Knowledge of guidelines set by agencies such as the Occupational Safety and Health Administration (OSHA), Clinical and Laboratory Standards Institute (CLSI), and the Centers for Disease Control and Prevention (CDC).
- Compliance: Understanding patient rights and confidentiality according to laws like the Health Insurance Portability and Accountability Act (HIPAA).

2. Patient Preparation (15% of the exam)

This section focuses on your ability to prepare patients for phlebotomy procedures. Topics include:

- Patient identification: Verification processes to ensure you're treating the correct patient.
- Education: Ability to explain the procedure to the patient and answer any questions.
- Collection equipment: Selection and preparation of appropriate collection equipment, including tubes, needles, and tourniquets.

3. Routine Blood Collections (30% of the exam)

As the largest component of the exam, this section tests your understanding and ability to carry out regular blood collection procedures. Topics include:

- Venipuncture: Knowledge of the proper technique for venipuncture, including finding suitable veins, appropriate insertion of the needle, and post-procedure care.

- Order of draw: Understanding of the correct order in which to fill blood collection tubes based on additives and the tests to be performed.
- Complications: Ability to identify and respond to complications during or after venipuncture, such as hematoma, syncope (fainting), or adverse patient reactions.

4. Special Collections (10% of the exam)

This segment assesses your knowledge of less common blood collection procedures. Topics include:

- Non-blood specimens: Collection of urine, stool, or swab specimens.
- Special blood collections: Collections such as blood cultures, glucose tolerance testing, and blood alcohol levels.
- Capillary puncture: Knowledge of proper fingerstick or heelstick procedures.

5. Point-of-Care Testing (10% of the exam)

This section focuses on your understanding of point-of-care testing procedures. Topics include:

- Glucose testing: Understanding of how to perform a point-of-care glucose test, including quality control checks.
- Other point-of-care tests: Familiarity with other potential point-of-care tests a phlebotomist might be required to perform, such as coagulation testing or hemoglobin/hematocrit testing.
- Quality control: Knowledge of how to ensure the accuracy and validity of point-of-care test results.

6. Processing and Handling of Specimens (20% of the exam)

The final section of the exam tests your understanding of what happens after specimen collection. Topics include:

- Transport: Proper labeling, handling, and transport of specimens to ensure their integrity.
- Processing: Understanding of how specimens are prepared for analysis, including centrifugation and aliquoting.
- Storage: Knowledge of proper storage conditions for various types of specimens.

Each of these six sections contains multiple-choice questions that will assess your understanding of the topics in depth. The exam is designed to ensure that Certified Phlebotomy Technicians have a well-rounded understanding of the role and can perform their duties to a high standard.

Section 1: Safety and Compliance:

Welcome to the first stepping stone in your journey to becoming a proficient Phlebotomy Technician - mastering Safety and Compliance. This section holds paramount importance, comprising 15% of the NHA CPT exam. It's crucial to not only your success in the exam but also your professional career in healthcare.

In the realm of phlebotomy, ensuring safety and adhering to regulatory compliance isn't an option - it's an absolute necessity. From the moment a patient walks into the lab until their specimen is analyzed, safety measures and compliance standards weave through each step.

Within Safety and Compliance, you'll delve into infection control protocols, grasp an understanding of safety regulations, and comprehend the essence of compliance.

Infection control is a significant part of maintaining safety. It ranges from routine practices such as hand hygiene to more specialized processes like the safe disposal of sharps and biohazardous waste. Mastering these steps ensures that you protect not just yourself, but also the patient and your colleagues from potential infection transmission.

Understanding safety regulations is vital. Guidelines set by institutions like the Occupational Safety and Health Administration (OSHA), the Clinical and Laboratory Standards Institute (CLSI), and the Centers for Disease Control and Prevention (CDC) form the bedrock of safety practices in phlebotomy. Familiarizing yourself with these regulations will help you to carry out procedures in a safe and efficient manner.

Lastly, we tackle compliance, which includes maintaining patient rights and confidentiality as stipulated by laws such as the Health Insurance Portability and Accountability Act (HIPAA). In this era of digital information, understanding how to handle patient information is of utmost importance.

Mastering the principles of safety and compliance is not merely about passing the exam. It's about laying a solid foundation for a career in phlebotomy where every action respects and safeguards the health and wellbeing of patients. As you explore this section, remember that these aren't just guidelines; they're a commitment to providing the highest quality of care in your role as a Phlebotomy Technician.

Let's turn the page and begin this vital journey into Safety and Compliance.

Standard Precautions are a set of infection control practices that aim to prevent transmission of diseases. Introduced by the Centers for Disease Control and Prevention (CDC), they are based on the principle that all blood, body fluids, secretions, excretions (except sweat), non-intact skin, and mucous membranes may contain transmissible infectious agents.

The key components of Standard Precautions include:

1. Hand Hygiene: This is considered one of the most effective ways to prevent the spread of infections. It includes washing hands with soap and water or using an alcohol-based hand sanitizer.

2. Use of Personal Protective Equipment (PPE): PPE, such as gloves, gowns, masks, and eye protection, is used to create a barrier between the healthcare worker and infectious agents.

3. Respiratory Hygiene/Cough Etiquette: This involves covering the mouth and nose during coughing or sneezing, using tissues or the elbow, followed by hand hygiene.

4. Safe Injection Practices: This includes using a new sterile syringe and needle for each injection and not sharing medication vials between patients.

5. Safe Handling of Potentially Contaminated Equipment or Surfaces in the Patient Environment: Regular cleaning and disinfection of the patient environment and reusable equipment is essential.

6. Sharps Safety: Safe handling and disposal of needles and other sharp instruments to prevent injuries that could lead to transmission of bloodborne pathogens.

Standard Precautions are vital in phlebotomy for several reasons. Firstly, they protect the phlebotomist from exposure to bloodborne pathogens, which is a significant risk given the nature of their work. Secondly, they protect patients from acquiring infections during the blood collection process. Lastly, they play a critical role in maintaining a safe and healthy environment in healthcare settings, protecting other healthcare workers and visitors. Thus, adherence to Standard Precautions is a fundamental aspect of quality healthcare delivery and patient safety.

When dealing with any healthcare procedure, especially phlebotomy, one cannot underestimate the value of properly utilizing Personal Protective Equipment (PPE). The sequence you follow when donning (putting on) and doffing (removing) PPE can significantly influence its effectiveness in protecting you from potential hazards.

Donning PPE
1. **Hand Hygiene**: Start by cleaning your hands with soap and water or an alcohol-based hand sanitizer. Hand hygiene is crucial to prevent the transfer of germs to the PPE you're about to put on.
2. **Gown**: After ensuring clean hands, put on a protective gown that covers your torso from neck to knees, your arms to the end of your wrists, and wraps around the back. Fasten at the back of the neck and waist.

3. **Mask or Respirator**: Next, place the mask over your nose, mouth, and chin. If it has ties, secure them at the crown of your head and base of your neck. If using a respirator, perform a user seal check to ensure a proper fit.
4. **Goggles or Face Shield**: Protect your eyes and face from splashes by wearing goggles or a face shield. Place the goggles over your eyes and adjust to fit. If you're wearing a face shield, it should fit over the front and sides of your face and past your chin.
5. **Gloves**: Last but not least, wear gloves that cover the cuffs (wrists) of the gown. Remember that gloves are single-use items.

Doffing PPE

Removing PPE is a process that requires careful attention to avoid contaminating yourself.

1. **Gloves**: Begin with your gloves. Grasp the outside of one glove at the wrist without touching your skin, then peel it off. Hold the removed glove in your gloved hand. Then, slide your ungloved fingers under the remaining glove at the wrist and peel it off over the first glove. Discard the gloves immediately into a waste container.
2. **Goggles or Face Shield**: Next, remove your eye protection by handling the ear or headpieces only. Once again, discard them right away if they are disposable or put reusable ones in the designated receptacle for cleaning.
3. **Gown**: Unfasten the gown ties and pull it away from your neck and shoulders. Be cautious to touch the inside of the gown only, then turn it inside out and roll it into a bundle. Dispose of it immediately in a waste container.
4. **Mask or Respirator**: Reach up to your face and touch only the ties or elastic band of the mask or respirator. Lift it away from your face and discard it, ensuring you don't touch the front of it.
5. **Hand Hygiene**: Finally, perform hand hygiene again with soap and water or alcohol-based hand sanitizer.

Remember, each step in this process is designed to safeguard your wellbeing and the health of your patients. Take the time to perfect these techniques and create an environment of safety and confidence.

Personal Protective Equipment (PPE), as the name suggests, is designed to protect healthcare personnel, including phlebotomists, from exposure to infectious agents and other hazards. Let's delve into the different types of PPE and when each is employed in a phlebotomy setting.

1. Gloves: Gloves are the most commonly used PPE in phlebotomy. They form a protective barrier between the phlebotomist and the patient, reducing the risk of transmitting infections. Gloves should be worn for every blood draw. They're typically made of latex, nitrile, or vinyl, with nitrile gloves being a common choice due to their puncture resistance and lack of allergenic proteins, which some people may react to in latex gloves.

2. Gowns: Gowns provide a barrier that protects clothing and skin from spills, sprays, or splashes of blood or body fluids. They're typically employed when a large amount of blood or other

potentially infectious materials is expected. An example might be during a difficult or prolonged blood draw.

3. Masks and Respirators: Masks protect the mouth and nose from droplets that may contain infectious agents. They're used during procedures that are likely to generate splashes or sprays of blood, body fluids, secretions, or excretions. A respirator, like an N95 mask, provides a higher level of protection and is used when airborne precautions are necessary.

4. Goggles and Face Shields: These protect the eyes, and in the case of face shields, the entire face, from splashes or sprays of blood or body fluids. Like masks, they're used when procedures have a high risk of generating splashes or sprays. Face shields have the added benefit of protecting the mask and preventing it from becoming wet, which can lower its effectiveness.

5. Caps and Shoe Covers: Although not commonly used in phlebotomy, caps and shoe covers can be used when there is a risk of contamination to the hair or shoes. This might be the case in certain specialty settings or when dealing with a large amount of blood or body fluids.

Remember, the purpose of PPE is to reduce the risk of exposure to infectious agents and other hazards. It is essential to use the correct type of PPE for each situation, but it's equally important to properly don and doff it to maintain its effectiveness and avoid self-contamination. Always keep in mind the vital role PPE plays in safeguarding your health, the health of your patients, and the overall safety of your work environment.

The use of Personal Protective Equipment (PPE) is paramount in healthcare settings like phlebotomy. However, when PPE is used improperly, it can pose numerous risks.

1. Cross-contamination: Perhaps the most significant hazard from improper use of PPE is cross-contamination, which can lead to the transmission of infectious agents. This can occur if PPE is not changed between patients or if contaminated PPE is touched with bare hands during removal.

2. Exposure to infectious agents: PPE that is not donned or doffed correctly can lead to exposure to bloodborne pathogens or other infectious materials. For example, removing gloves incorrectly could result in the hands coming into contact with the outside of the gloves, which may be contaminated.

3. Allergic reactions: Some people are allergic to latex, which is used in certain types of gloves. Wearing latex gloves can cause allergic reactions in these individuals, ranging from skin irritation to more severe responses like difficulty breathing.

4. Physical injuries: Improper use of PPE can also result in physical injuries. For instance, not wearing gloves can expose the skin to needlestick injuries, while not wearing eye protection can risk injuries from splashes of blood or other body fluids.

To prevent these hazards, healthcare professionals can adhere to the following practices:

1. Correct usage of PPE: Always follow proper procedures for donning and doffing PPE. This includes hand hygiene before and after using PPE, putting on and removing PPE in the correct order, and avoiding touching the front of potentially contaminated PPE during removal.

2. Regular training and updates: Regular training and refresher courses can ensure that all healthcare workers are up-to-date on the correct use of PPE. This should include training on the selection of appropriate PPE for different situations.

3. Use of hypoallergenic alternatives: For individuals allergic to latex, hypoallergenic alternatives like nitrile or vinyl gloves can be used.

4. Compliance with infection prevention protocols: Besides PPE, following other infection prevention protocols, such as standard precautions and hand hygiene, can further reduce the risk of transmission of infectious agents.

In sum, while PPE plays a crucial role in protecting healthcare workers and patients from infectious agents, improper use can result in various hazards. Through proper use and adherence to infection prevention protocols, these hazards can be effectively mitigated.

Let's dive deep into the topic of safety and infection control in phlebotomy, starting with its significance.

Safety and infection control are at the heart of any phlebotomy procedure. With the nature of the job requiring direct contact with patients and their bodily fluids, there's a considerable risk of transmitting infections between patients and healthcare workers. Proper safety procedures protect not only the phlebotomist but also the patients from potential harm, making these measures an integral part of patient care.

Now, this leads us to Standard Precautions, a set of infection control practices designed to prevent the transmission of diseases in any healthcare setting. They apply to all patient care, regardless of suspected or confirmed infection status of the patient, and they revolve around treating all blood and bodily fluids (except sweat) as potentially infectious. Standard Precautions involve practices such as hand hygiene, use of PPE, respiratory hygiene, and safe injection practices, to name a few.

Personal Protective Equipment (PPE) comes as one of the critical components of Standard Precautions. These are barriers used to protect skin, clothing, mucous membranes, and the respiratory system from infectious agents. In phlebotomy, the appropriate use of gloves, gowns, masks, goggles, or face shields, depending on the situation, forms a crucial line of defense against the transmission of diseases.

Another major aspect of safety in phlebotomy is the handling and disposal of sharps. Phlebotomists frequently handle needles, lancets, and other sharp objects, which can potentially lead to injuries and exposure to bloodborne pathogens. Essential steps for the safe handling of sharps include never recapping used needles, using a one-handed scoop technique if recapping is necessary, immediately disposing of used sharps in a puncture-resistant sharps container, and handling sharps with care to prevent accidental injuries.

In this context, quality assurance surfaces as a critical component of phlebotomy. It refers to the systematic monitoring and evaluation of various aspects of a project, service, or facility to ensure standards of quality are being met. It aims to prevent errors, promote accurate test results, and ensure patient satisfaction. From the phlebotomist's technique to the condition of the equipment, quality assurance encompasses all aspects of the phlebotomy process.

The implementation of quality control in a phlebotomy setting typically involves regular equipment checks, reviewing procedures and technique, continuing education for staff, and regular performance evaluations. Regular audits and review of adverse events also contribute to this process.

Documentation and reporting form an integral part of quality assurance and control procedures. They ensure transparency and offer a medium to evaluate and improve services based on past experiences. Accurate documentation, including patient identification, tests performed, test results, and any issues or deviations from standard procedure, can help to prevent errors and improve the overall quality of care.

Moving onto legal, professional, and ethical standards, patients have a legal right to privacy and confidentiality. It's the responsibility of healthcare workers to protect this right by keeping all health-related information confidential, sharing it only when necessary for the provision of care or when legally required.

Consent is another crucial legal concept in phlebotomy. Before drawing blood, the phlebotomist must obtain consent from the patient or their legal representative. This process involves explaining the procedure, including its risks and benefits, and verifying the patient's identity using at least two identifiers, such as the patient's name and date of birth.

Lastly, professional conduct in phlebotomy revolves around respecting each patient's rights and dignity, providing competent care, maintaining personal and professional integrity, and working within the individual phlebotomist's scope of practice. A phlebotomist's scope of practice includes tasks like drawing blood, preparing samples for testing, following infection control and safety procedures, and providing patient education and support, but it doesn't include interpreting test results or providing medical advice.

So, we've covered a lot, and it's important to remember that these are just the broad strokes. Each topic here is rich with detail, but with thorough study and practice, you'll master these skills and concepts. They form the foundation of safe and effective phlebotomy practice, and each one is integral to your success as a phlebotomist.

The concept of Standard Precautions is fundamental in any healthcare setting, including phlebotomy. Initially developed by the Centers for Disease Control and Prevention (CDC), Standard Precautions serve as a key strategy for infection prevention and control.

These precautions are essentially a set of guidelines that assume blood and various body fluids from any patient could potentially harbor infectious agents. Therefore, they prescribe the most effective methods for preventing the spread of pathogens in healthcare settings, irrespective of the patient's disease status or diagnosis.

The components of Standard Precautions encompass several crucial elements:

Hand Hygiene: This is perhaps the most effective way to prevent the spread of infections. Healthcare workers should clean their hands before and after each patient encounter, after touching blood, body fluids, secretions, excretions, and contaminated items, even if gloves are worn.
Use of Personal Protective Equipment (PPE): The use of PPE such as gloves, gowns, masks, and eye protection is advised based on anticipated exposure. For example, gloves should be worn when it's likely the hands will touch blood, body fluids, or potentially contaminated surfaces.
Respiratory Hygiene and Cough Etiquette: Patients should be educated on covering the mouth and nose during sneezing or coughing, using tissues or elbow instead of hands, and disposing of tissues correctly.
Patient Care Equipment: Proper cleaning, disinfection, and sterilization of patient care equipment are essential to prevent the spread of infectious agents.
Safe Injection Practices: These practices aim to prevent transmission of infectious diseases between one patient and another, or between a patient and healthcare provider during preparation and administration of parenteral medications.
Safe Handling of Potentially Contaminated Laundry: Healthcare workers must handle, transport, and process used linen in a manner that prevents skin and mucous membrane exposures, contamination of clothing, and transfer of pathogens to other patients or the environment.
Adherence to these precautions helps ensure a safer environment for patients and healthcare personnel alike. However, the effectiveness of Standard Precautions is largely dependent on

individual healthcare workers understanding these principles and putting them into practice consistently.

The safe handling and disposal of sharps in a healthcare setting is a non-negotiable, key part of maintaining patient and worker safety. Sharps include any objects that can prick, cut, or puncture the skin, such as needles, scalpels, lancets, and broken glass. They can potentially carry bloodborne pathogens, posing a significant risk for healthcare professionals, especially phlebotomists.

Follow these essential steps for the safe handling and disposal of sharps:

1. **Never Recap Used Needles:** After use, needles should never be recapped, bent, broken, or manipulated by hand. Recapping needles can lead to accidental puncture injuries, which can potentially transmit infections.
2. **Immediate Disposal:** Sharps should be disposed of immediately after use in a puncture-resistant, leak-proof, and labeled or color-coded container. These sharps disposal containers should be readily accessible in the area where sharps are being used.
3. **Correct Disposal Container:** Always dispose of sharps in containers that are specially designed for them. They should be sturdy and sealable to prevent any sharps from sticking out or falling out.
4. **Don't Overfill Disposal Container:** Sharps disposal containers should not be filled beyond the marked fill line. Overfilling can lead to accidents during disposal.
5. **Safe Transportation:** When a sharps container becomes full, it should be closed securely to prevent spillage, and it should be transported carefully to the disposal area.
6. **Proper Training:** All healthcare workers should be properly trained in the safe handling and disposal of sharps. This includes knowledge of the potential hazards and the use of protective equipment.
7. **Emergency Protocols:** In case of a sharps injury, there should be clear protocols in place to ensure immediate and appropriate action.

Remember, maintaining safety while handling sharps isn't just about protecting yourself, but also about preserving the safety and health of your colleagues and patients. These steps are part of the Standard Precautions that every healthcare worker, especially phlebotomists, should know and follow.

Quality assurance is a fundamental aspect of any healthcare practice, and phlebotomy is no exception. Phlebotomy, which involves drawing blood from patients for various diagnostic tests, can greatly influence a patient's diagnostic journey and subsequent treatment plan. Therefore, the assurance of quality in every step of the process is crucial.

Quality assurance in phlebotomy focuses on ensuring accurate test results by minimizing pre-analytical errors. These errors could arise during patient identification, specimen collection, handling, transportation, or processing. By implementing strict quality assurance protocols, phlebotomists ensure that each patient receives the correct diagnosis based on accurate and reliable test results, contributing to more effective patient care.

Quality assurance also emphasizes the importance of patient safety and comfort during the phlebotomy procedure. It ensures that phlebotomists follow safe and ethical practices, minimizing the risk of cross-contamination or infection and ensuring the patient's comfort during the procedure.

On the other hand, quality control in a phlebotomy setting refers to the specific procedures used to ensure the quality of the test results. It involves the regular maintenance and calibration of equipment used for blood collection and testing, monitoring the accuracy and precision of test results through control samples, and maintaining the competency of the staff through continuous education and performance evaluations.

The implementation of quality control in phlebotomy involves various steps, including:

1. **Equipment Control:** Regular checks and calibration of equipment used for blood collection are done to ensure they are functioning optimally.
2. **Reagent Control:** The reagents used for testing should be stored properly and checked for their expiry dates. They should be discarded if found to be expired or contaminated.
3. **Control Samples:** These are samples with known values that are tested alongside patient samples. If the results from control samples fall within the predetermined range, it indicates that the test system is working accurately.
4. **Proficiency Testing:** This involves testing samples provided by an external organization to verify the accuracy of test results.
5. **Continuous Education and Training:** Regular training and updating of staff on new methods, protocols, or guidelines are critical to maintaining a high level of competency in phlebotomy procedures.

In essence, quality assurance and quality control go hand in hand in ensuring that patients receive the most accurate diagnosis and the best care, which are the primary goals of any healthcare practice.

Documentation and reporting are essential components in quality assurance (QA) and quality control (QC) procedures within phlebotomy and healthcare at large. They provide a written record of all activities, enabling traceability, transparency, and accountability in the phlebotomy process.

Accurate and timely documentation serves as an evidence-based approach to confirm that all steps in the phlebotomy process - from patient identification and sample collection to processing, testing, and disposal - were executed correctly and safely. It also records that the instruments and equipment were properly maintained and calibrated, and all relevant standard operating procedures were adhered to.

Documentation assists in the monitoring of performance over time. Regular audits of these documents can identify patterns, trends, or deviations from standard protocols, signaling areas that may need improvement. For example, if it's noted that errors often occur during a particular time or shift, actions can be taken to address the underlying issues, such as additional staff training or revising shift schedules.

Reporting, on the other hand, is a mechanism to communicate information from these records to relevant stakeholders. Reports provide a synopsis of operations, outlining successes and areas needing improvement. This communication can guide decision-making, policy development, and ensure that all staff members are aware of the current state of affairs, thereby maintaining a high standard of service.

In quality control, documentation and reporting help confirm that internal controls (including proficiency testing and control samples) are in place and functioning as expected. They also provide evidence that any identified issues were addressed appropriately, and corrective actions were taken to prevent their recurrence.

Furthermore, in the event of an error or adverse event, detailed documentation can provide a clear understanding of the circumstances leading to the incident, supporting a thorough investigation and the development of appropriate corrective actions.

Overall, documentation and reporting function as critical tools for continual improvement, supporting the ultimate goal of quality assurance and control: to ensure the highest standards of patient care and safety.

Legal rights of patients, especially in relation to confidentiality, are cornerstones of healthcare practice, including phlebotomy. They are ingrained within the ethical code of conduct and legal frameworks that regulate the healthcare industry.

In the realm of phlebotomy, these rights entail many dimensions:

Informed Consent: Patients have the right to be informed about the purpose, benefits, risks, and alternatives to a phlebotomy procedure before it is performed. They are entitled to grant or deny consent based on this information. This consent can be withdrawn at any time.

Privacy: Patients have the right to privacy during the phlebotomy procedure. Phlebotomists should always ensure they conduct the procedure in a private, non-public area and take necessary steps to minimize exposure.

Confidentiality: Information related to a patient's health status, diagnosis, prognosis, and treatment, as well as personal identifiers, should remain confidential. This means that such data can only be shared with authorized individuals involved in patient care, or as otherwise required by law.

Security of Health Records: With the advent of digital health records, it's vital to safeguard the data from unauthorized access, modification, disclosure, or destruction, whether accidental or deliberate.

Respect and Dignity: Every patient deserves to be treated with respect, dignity, and non-discrimination. This includes sensitivity to their cultural, religious, and personal beliefs and practices.

Confidentiality in phlebotomy, as in all healthcare professions, is crucial for several reasons:

Trust: Confidentiality is fundamental in building trust between the patient and the healthcare provider. Patients will be more open about their health status if they believe their information will be kept confidential.

Ethics and Legal Requirements: Confidentiality is not only an ethical obligation but also a legal requirement under laws such as the Health Insurance Portability and Accountability Act (HIPAA) in the U.S. Non-compliance with these regulations can lead to serious legal consequences for both the individual and the institution.

Patient Well-being: Respect for confidentiality can help to alleviate patient anxiety, increase their satisfaction, and ultimately lead to improved health outcomes.

So, as a phlebotomist, maintaining patient rights and upholding confidentiality isn't merely a regulatory or ethical obligation - it's a fundamental aspect of high-quality patient care.

In phlebotomy, as in all medical procedures, consent is the agreement or permission given by the patient for the procedure to be carried out. It is based on the principle of patient autonomy and informed decision-making. For consent to be valid, it must be informed, voluntary, and given by an individual who is competent.

Informed consent in phlebotomy involves explaining to the patient about the procedure, why it is being done, what it will involve, its benefits, and any associated risks or discomfort. This way, the patient understands what they are agreeing to, which allows them to make an informed decision about their care.

It is worth noting that consent can be expressed (verbally or in writing) or implied (through actions). For example, a patient extending their arm for venipuncture can be seen as giving implied consent. However, for certain procedures or circumstances, written and explicit verbal consent may be required.

Patient identification is a crucial part of the consent process. Proper identification ensures that the correct procedure is performed on the correct patient. This involves asking the patient to confirm their identity, typically their full name and date of birth, and comparing it with the information on the lab requisition form and specimen label. The phlebotomist should do this before obtaining consent and before starting the procedure. This double-check helps prevent identification errors, which are a common type of error in phlebotomy and laboratory medicine.

In summary, consent and patient identification are fundamental steps in the pre-analytical phase of phlebotomy, playing a pivotal role in patient safety, ethical practice, and reduction of errors in laboratory medicine.

Professional conduct in phlebotomy encompasses a broad range of behaviors and attitudes expected from a healthcare professional. To be proficient, a phlebotomist must display a fusion of technical skills, interpersonal communication abilities, and a firm grasp of ethical guidelines.

Professionalism begins with personal attributes, including empathy, respect, and cultural sensitivity. Patients should always be treated with kindness and courtesy. A phlebotomist should listen to patients' concerns and questions, provide reassurances when needed, and ensure patients' dignity is upheld at all times.

Equally important is communication. Phlebotomists must be able to convey important information about the procedure to patients effectively and should maintain an open line of communication with the rest of the healthcare team to ensure accurate and timely diagnostic results.

Professional conduct also demands that phlebotomists adhere to ethical principles. This includes maintaining confidentiality, obtaining informed consent before the procedure, and respecting patients' rights to refuse treatment.

In terms of scope of practice, phlebotomists primarily draw blood for diagnostic testing. This includes venipunctures and capillary punctures. They may also process specimens and prepare them for laboratory testing. However, phlebotomists are not involved in the actual diagnostic analysis of blood specimens; this is the domain of laboratory technicians and clinical laboratory scientists.

Additionally, the phlebotomist's role extends to patient education, infection control, and safety procedures. It's crucial that phlebotomists understand the boundaries of their role and do not step beyond them - for instance, they must not interpret test results for patients, as this falls under the physician's purview.

In essence, a phlebotomist is an integral part of the healthcare team, with a unique set of responsibilities that require a blend of technical know-how, interpersonal skill, and ethical discernment.

Section 2: Patient Preparation:

As we delve into the second part of our journey, Section 2: Patient Preparation, we stand on the cusp of two realms: the safety procedures we've left behind and the compassionate, patient-centric approach we're about to embrace. In this section, we shall shed light on the essential and subtle art of preparing patients for phlebotomy procedures.

Here, we'll take a closer look at the critical initial steps that lay the groundwork for the entire phlebotomy process. From patient identification to the importance of informed consent, from patient positioning to the selection of the appropriate site for venipuncture, each aspect requires meticulous attention to detail and a patient-first attitude.

But patient preparation is more than just these technical steps. It also involves the invaluable skill of effective communication, facilitating a supportive and reassuring environment, and educating patients about the procedure. After all, a relaxed and cooperative patient often leads to a smoother, more efficient procedure.

As we traverse this section, remember that each patient is unique, bringing their own set of experiences, concerns, and expectations. A skilled phlebotomist is an adaptable one, able to meet each patient where they are and guide them through the procedure with empathy and expertise.

Buckle up, and let's dive into the intricacies of patient preparation in phlebotomy!

Patient identification is a fundamental procedure in phlebotomy and healthcare in general. A slip in the identification process can lead to grave errors such as incorrect diagnosis, treatment, and data recording. In the practical setting, the process involves the following steps:
1. **Verification of Patient Details:** The phlebotomist should verify the patient's full name, date of birth, and any other necessary identifiers such as the medical record number or patient ID number. This information should match with what is on the test requisition form and the patient's wristband if one is present. Always ask the patient to spell out their name instead of confirming with a yes/no question. For instance, ask, "Can you spell your last name?" instead of "Is your last name Johnson?"
2. **Use of Identification Bands:** In most healthcare facilities, patients are required to wear identification bands that contain essential information such as their name, date of birth, and a unique identifying number. Before any procedure, phlebotomists must check these bands for confirmation.
3. **Verification from Patient:** A patient who is conscious and competent should confirm their identity verbally. This is generally considered the most reliable method of identification.

4. **Check the Test Requisition Form:** It is also important to double-check the details on the test requisition form to ensure that it matches the information given by the patient and the information on the identification band.

Remember, these steps are not optional and must be strictly adhered to. The accurate identification of patients is a standard procedure designed to prevent errors in patient care. Patient identification is so crucial that it is considered the primary standard in the National Patient Safety Goals established by The Joint Commission, an organization that accredits healthcare organizations in the United States.

Phlebotomy, like any other medical procedure, requires accurate patient identification to ensure that the correct person receives the appropriate care. Here are the best practices in the context of phlebotomy:

1. **Two-Factor Identification:** Always verify at least two identifying factors, which typically include the patient's name and date of birth. These details should be cross-checked with the information available on the patient's identification band and requisition form.
2. **Direct Patient Verification:** The most reliable identification source is the patient themselves. When the patient is conscious and competent, always ask them to provide their name and date of birth.
3. **Requisition Form Matching:** Cross-check the identification data with the information on the requisition form. If you spot any discrepancies, do not proceed with the procedure until you've clarified and resolved the discrepancy.
4. **Identity Band Confirmation:** Identity bands are commonly used in healthcare settings. Before phlebotomy, ensure the name, date of birth, and any additional identification numbers on the band match with the requisition form and the patient's verbal confirmation.
5. **Speak Up Culture:** Encourage patients to speak up if they notice that the information on their wristband or in their records is incorrect, or if they haven't been asked for their identification.
6. **Double Checking:** If there are any doubts or discrepancies, double-check with another healthcare professional. It's better to spend a bit more time in verification than risk a misidentification error.
7. **Patient Unconscious or Non-communicative:** In case the patient is unconscious or unable to communicate, use medical records and identification bands for identification. If there's no ID band, follow your institution's guidelines for such situations.

The primary goal is to ensure patient safety, so these best practices are designed to minimize errors. Remember, identification errors can have serious consequences, including wrong-person procedures, misdiagnoses, and incorrect treatment plans, all of which can be potentially life-threatening.

Indeed, errors during the patient identification process can lead to several complications, some of which are truly serious. Here are some common mistakes and their potential ramifications:

1. **Misidentification:** This is the most common and serious error where the patient is mistaken for another. It can occur due to similarities in names, incorrect entry of patient information, or misreading the identity band. This mistake can lead to wrong-person procedures, causing harmful or even lethal consequences.
2. **Reliance on Room or Bed Number:** Patients can be moved around for various reasons within a healthcare facility, so relying on the room or bed number instead of directly identifying the patient can lead to mistakes.
3. **Assuming Identity Based on Diagnosis or Age:** It's incorrect and unsafe to identify a patient based on their diagnosis, age, or any other factor not specific to them. This could lead to harmful mix-ups.
4. **Not Confirming Identity with Patient:** Not involving the patient in their identification, when they are conscious and competent, can increase the risk of misidentification.
5. **Inadequate Verification in Urgent Situations:** During emergencies, the identification process can sometimes be rushed, but even in urgent situations, proper identification should not be compromised.
6. **Lack of Standardized Identification Methods:** If the healthcare setting doesn't have a standardized identification procedure, it can lead to inconsistent practices and increase the risk of errors.

Consequences of these errors are serious and far-reaching. Misidentification can lead to incorrect blood transfusion, wrong-site surgery, wrong-person procedure, medication errors, and incorrect patient orders. These mistakes not only put the patient's safety and health at risk but also increase the liability for the healthcare professionals and the institution.

In order to prevent these errors, it's crucial to adhere to standardized identification procedures, double-check information, and involve the patient in the identification process whenever possible. Remember, patient safety is the ultimate priority.

Preventing patient identification errors and rectifying them should they occur is a top priority in phlebotomy. Here are a few strategies that can be implemented:
1. **Double-Check Patient Details:** Always verify the patient's identity by using at least two identifiers. This can include the patient's full name, date of birth, or an assigned identification number. If the patient is conscious, confirm their identity by asking them directly.
2. **Use Standardized Patient Identification Systems:** Implementing a consistent and standardized patient identification system can significantly reduce errors. This may include barcoded wristbands, electronic verification systems, or other technology designed for patient identification.
3. **Staff Training:** Regularly training staff on the importance of accurate patient identification and on correct identification procedures can help reduce errors. Encourage staff to be vigilant and not rush the identification process, even in urgent situations.
4. **Involve the Patient:** Whenever possible, involve the patient in the identification process. Ask them to confirm their name and other relevant details.

5. **Correcting Mistakes:** If a mistake occurs, it's essential to rectify it immediately. Update any incorrect patient details in the system, inform the relevant healthcare providers about the error, and make sure the correct information is passed on to all staff involved in the patient's care.

6. **Open Communication:** Foster a culture of open communication where staff feel comfortable reporting identification errors or near misses without fear of punishment. Learning from mistakes can provide valuable insight into potential weaknesses in the system and can help prevent future errors.

7. **Regular Audits:** Regularly audit patient identification processes and procedures to identify any potential issues or areas for improvement. Make necessary adjustments based on audit findings to continually improve patient safety.

By implementing these measures, phlebotomists can significantly reduce the likelihood of patient identification errors and improve overall patient safety and care.

There's quite an assortment of equipment used in phlebotomy, each serving a distinct purpose. Here are some of the most common ones:

1. **Needles:** These are the primary tools used to puncture veins for blood collection. They come in various sizes, typically 20-23 gauge for adults and 23-25 gauge for children or for capillary punctures.

2. **Evacuated Collection Tubes:** These vacuum-sealed tubes draw in a predetermined volume of blood once the vein is punctured. The tubes often have additives in them that either cause the blood to clot or prevent clotting, depending on the tests to be performed.

3. **Tourniquets:** These are used to apply pressure to the upper arm, making the veins more prominent and easier to access.

4. **Tube Holders or Adapters:** These are plastic devices that hold the collection tube in place during blood collection.

5. **Lancets:** These are used for capillary punctures, such as fingersticks or heelsticks.

6. **Alcohol Wipes:** Used to clean the puncture site before the collection procedure.

7. **Gauze and Bandages:** After the blood draw, these are used to stop any bleeding and cover the puncture site.

8. **Sharps Container:** A puncture-proof and leak-proof container used for the safe disposal of used needles and lancets.

9. **Gloves:** PPE (Personal Protective Equipment) to protect the phlebotomist and patient from cross-contamination.

10. **Centrifuge:** A machine used to separate the components of the blood after collection for certain types of tests.

11. **Blood Collection Tray or Cart:** Holds all the necessary equipment for the blood draw, keeping everything organized and readily accessible.

These items collectively allow a phlebotomist to perform blood draws safely and efficiently, all while maximizing comfort for the patient.

Choosing the right phlebotomy equipment is vital for both the patient's safety and the success of the blood draw. Here are some key factors to consider:

1. **Patient's Age and Size:** Pediatric patients, for example, have smaller veins, so a smaller gauge needle and a lancet might be appropriate for them. Similarly, elderly patients may have fragile or difficult-to-access veins, requiring a careful choice of equipment.
2. **Patient's Health Condition:** Certain medical conditions can affect the veins and blood collection. For instance, patients with hematoma or venous thrombosis might require a different approach, and patients on blood thinners may bleed more, necessitating extra gauze or bandages.
3. **Volume of Blood Needed:** The required volume of blood for the test(s) being conducted will influence the choice of collection tubes and possibly the needle size.
4. **Site of Venipuncture:** Not all veins can accommodate all sizes of needles. The choice of the needle will also depend on the chosen venipuncture site.
5. **Purpose of the Draw:** If you are collecting blood cultures, you may need specific bottles. If you are testing for glucose levels, you'll need tubes with an anticoagulant and a glycolytic inhibitor.
6. **Patient Comfort:** Some patients might be afraid of larger needles, in which case you might opt for a smaller one if possible. Additionally, certain tourniquets might be more comfortable for the patient than others.
7. **Professional Comfort and Experience:** Ultimately, phlebotomists should use equipment they are comfortable and experienced with. It's important to use equipment that allows for the most efficient and effective draw.

By carefully considering these factors, phlebotomists can ensure they use the most suitable equipment for each individual patient and situation, ensuring high-quality samples for accurate testing.

Effective communication is pivotal in any healthcare setting, and phlebotomy is no exception. The phlebotomy process can be daunting for some patients, so clear and empathetic communication can alleviate anxieties, facilitate cooperation, and ultimately enhance the success of the blood draw.

Here are a few critical communication skills phlebotomists should aim to develop:

1. **Active Listening:** Pay attention to what the patient is saying and respond appropriately. If a patient is anxious, try to address their concerns. If they mention a health condition that could affect the draw, take that into account.
2. **Clear Explanation:** Clearly explain each step of the process to the patient. Many people are afraid of the unknown, so knowledge of what to expect can provide comfort.
3. **Patience:** Some patients may require additional time to understand the procedure or may need information repeated. Being patient and accommodating can enhance the patient's comfort and compliance.
4. **Empathy:** Acknowledge the patient's feelings and provide reassurance. Phrases like "I understand that you're nervous, many people feel that way. I'm here to make sure this goes as smoothly as possible for you" can go a long way.

5. **Non-verbal Communication:** Maintain eye contact when speaking, use open body language, and consider your facial expressions. These cues can convey empathy and respect.
6. **Interpersonal Skills:** Building rapport with the patient can help them feel more comfortable and cooperative. A friendly demeanor and a bit of small talk can make the experience less clinical and impersonal.
7. **Professional Language:** Use appropriate medical terminology with colleagues but avoid overly technical language with patients, which could be confusing or intimidating.
8. **Cultural Competency:** Be aware of cultural differences in communication and adjust your approach accordingly.

By honing these skills, a phlebotomist can improve their interactions with patients, leading to a smoother and more positive experience for all involved.

Ensuring patient comfort throughout the phlebotomy procedure is crucial. It not only humanizes the healthcare experience, but it can also facilitate cooperation and potentially improve results. Here are some ways a phlebotomist can ensure patient comfort:

Before the Procedure:
1. **Patient education:** Explain the process clearly and answer any questions the patient may have. This can help reduce anxiety and establish trust.
2. **Active listening:** Pay attention to the patient's verbal and nonverbal cues. If they express fear or discomfort, acknowledge their feelings and offer reassurance.
3. **Preparation:** Ensure that all equipment is ready before beginning, to minimize the time the patient spends waiting in anxiety.

During the Procedure:
4. **Gentle touch:** Use a gentle touch while securing the vein and inserting the needle.
5. **Distraction:** Engage the patient in light conversation to divert their attention from the procedure. You can also suggest they focus on a point in the room or on their breathing.
6. **Pain management:** Use a local anesthetic, if necessary and appropriate, to reduce discomfort.

After the Procedure:
7. **Post-procedure care:** Inform the patient about aftercare, such as applying pressure to the site, leaving the bandage on for a certain amount of time, and recognizing signs of complications.
8. **Express gratitude:** Thank the patient for their cooperation. A little gratitude can go a long way in making a patient feel valued and comfortable.

In terms of distraction techniques, conversation is often the most effective. Discussing neutral topics, like the weather or recent local events, can divert attention from the procedure. Asking open-ended questions about the patient's interests or hobbies can also help.

For children, tactics may involve visual distractions like toys, books, or videos, or involving the child in a simple game. Regardless of the specific technique, the key is to be attentive and responsive to each patient's individual needs and preferences.

The choice of venipuncture site is guided by a sound understanding of human anatomy and physiology, particularly the circulatory system.

Blood in the human body is primarily transported via an intricate network of blood vessels, including arteries, veins, and capillaries. However, for phlebotomy purposes, we focus on veins as these are the sites of blood collection. The veins are less sensitive as compared to arteries and are closer to the surface of the skin, making them ideal for venipuncture.

Key sites for venipuncture include the antecubital area (the area of the arm in front of the elbow) and the top of the hand. The antecubital area is generally preferred because it has three significant veins: the median cubital vein, the cephalic vein, and the basilic vein. The median cubital vein, located in the middle of the antecubital area, is typically the first choice for blood collection because it is usually the most prominent and accessible vein.

However, the specific site selection depends on factors such as the patient's comfort, vein condition (size, depth, direction, and condition), the type and volume of specimen required, and the phlebotomist's experience. For example, if the median cubital vein is not suitable or is inaccessible, the cephalic vein (located laterally in the arm and is the second-largest vein) or the basilic vein (located medially and is often deeper and less stable) can be chosen.

In some instances, especially when dealing with patients with difficult veins, phlebotomists might need to resort to other veins, such as those on the dorsal side of the hand or lower arm. However, these are usually the last resort due to higher chances of patient discomfort and complications. In such cases, a good understanding of peripheral veins' anatomy outside the antecubital area becomes essential.

In sum, a sound understanding of the human circulatory system, primarily focusing on veins' anatomy and physiology, is crucial in selecting the most suitable site for venipuncture.

Selecting the optimal site for venipuncture is a crucial aspect of the phlebotomy process, and it involves several important considerations:
1. **Patient's Age and Condition**: The patient's age, overall health, and specific medical condition can influence site selection. For instance, in elderly patients or those with fragile veins, the veins in the antecubital area may be difficult to locate or prone to damage during the venipuncture.
2. **Vein Condition**: A good vein for venipuncture is usually large, palpable, visible, and resilient when depressed and refilled rapidly when released. It should not be sclerosed or thrombosed. The vein should be straight or have a gentle curve for an easier and safer blood draw.
3. **Patient Comfort**: The chosen site should be as comfortable as possible for the patient. This consideration includes avoiding areas with bruises, scars, rashes, or any visible sign of infection.

4. **Quantity of Blood Needed**: The volume of blood required for testing can also influence the choice of venipuncture site. A larger vein can accommodate a larger volume of blood without collapsing.
5. **Previous Venipunctures**: Try to avoid areas that have been recently used for venipuncture to prevent unnecessary pain or injury to the patient.

In most adult patients, the first choice for venipuncture is the median cubital vein in the antecubital fossa due to its size and accessibility. If this site is not viable, other choices may include the cephalic vein or basilic vein in the same area, or veins in the hand or wrist. The choice of site also needs to take into account any relevant clinical guidelines or institutional policies.

Identifying unsuitable sites for venipuncture is a crucial aspect of ensuring patient safety and the integrity of the collected specimen. Several signs may indicate that a particular site is unsuitable:

1. **Thrombosed or Sclerosed Veins**: Thrombosed veins have blood clots within them, making them dangerous for venipuncture. Sclerosed veins are hard and cord-like due to scarring or disease and are typically difficult to penetrate, which could lead to failed venipuncture.
2. **Inflamed or Infected Skin**: If the skin overlying a vein is red, swollen, hot, or shows signs of an active infection, it should be avoided to prevent spreading the infection or causing additional discomfort to the patient.
3. **Bruised or Hematoma Sites**: These sites are often painful and may indicate damage to the vein or surrounding tissues.
4. **Areas with Intravenous Lines or Medical Devices**: These areas are often not suitable for venipuncture to avoid disturbing the devices and to reduce the risk of infection.
5. **Arms on the Side of Mastectomy**: For patients who have undergone a mastectomy, it's important not to perform venipuncture on the side of the surgery to prevent lymphedema.
6. **Areas with Edema**: Excessive fluid accumulation may make it difficult to locate the vein and could also dilute the blood sample.

Choosing an unsuitable site for venipuncture can result in several potential risks. These include patient discomfort or pain, injury to the vein or surrounding tissues, poor quality or inadequate volume of the blood sample, and a heightened risk of complications such as infection, phlebitis (inflammation of the vein), hematoma, or nerve damage. Therefore, a thorough assessment of potential venipuncture sites is key to ensuring a safe and successful procedure.

Preparing a venipuncture site involves a few critical steps that ensure the safety and success of the procedure. These steps are as follows:

1. **Assess the Patient**: Before the actual procedure, ask the patient about any allergies, particularly to antiseptics or latex. Also, inquire about any previous experiences with blood draws, especially if there have been difficulties or complications.

2. **Choose the Site**: The next step is to choose an appropriate venipuncture site, typically in the antecubital area where the veins are most accessible. Make sure to assess the vein's condition by palpating for size, direction, and resilience.

3. **Clean the Site**: The selected site should then be cleaned with an appropriate antiseptic, such as 70% isopropyl alcohol or chlorhexidine, depending on your facility's protocol. Clean in a circular motion from the center of the site outwards. This step helps to minimize the risk of infection.

4. **Allow to Dry**: This is a crucial step that's often overlooked. The antiseptic should be allowed to dry completely to ensure its effectiveness and to minimize discomfort when the needle is inserted. It's important not to blow on the site, wave hands over it, or use gauze to speed up the drying process, as these actions could introduce bacteria.

5. **Put on Gloves**: Once the site is dry, put on a new pair of gloves. This is to protect both the phlebotomist and the patient.

6. **Prepare Equipment**: While the site is drying, you can use this time to prepare the necessary equipment such as the needle, holder, and blood collection tubes.

7. **Apply Tourniquet**: A tourniquet should be applied 3-4 inches above the venipuncture site to make the veins more prominent. However, the tourniquet should not be left on for more than 1 minute to avoid hemoconcentration, which could alter test results.

8. **Reassess the Vein**: After applying the tourniquet, reassess the chosen vein by palpating it. The vein should feel soft and bouncy. If it feels hard or cord-like, another site should be chosen.

After these steps, the venipuncture site is ready for the blood draw procedure. It's essential to keep communicating with the patient throughout this process, explaining each step, and ensuring they are comfortable and prepared for the venipuncture.

Section 3: Routine Blood Collections:

Welcome to Section 3: Routine Blood Collections. In this section, we delve into the heart of phlebotomy practice—the collection of blood samples. From understanding the different blood collection tubes and their uses, to performing the venipuncture procedure, we will explore all facets of routine blood collection, with an emphasis on ensuring patient safety and comfort.

Topics covered in this section are as follows.

Understanding Blood Collection Tubes and Their Uses - In this chapter, we will identify the different types of blood collection tubes used in phlebotomy, their additives, the tests associated with them, and the importance of the order of draw.

The Venipuncture Procedure - This chapter provides a step-by-step guide to the venipuncture procedure. We will discuss how to assemble the necessary supplies, perform the venipuncture safely and effectively, and handle any potential complications.

Complications and Special Considerations - Here, we will delve into potential complications during blood collection and discuss special considerations for patients with difficult veins, those experiencing anxiety or fear, and pediatric or geriatric patients.

Post-Venipuncture Procedure and Patient Care - The final chapter covers what happens after the blood draw, including sample handling and processing, post-venipuncture patient care, and how to handle adverse events such as syncope.

By the end of this section, you'll be equipped with a thorough understanding of the routine blood collection process, including both the practical and interpersonal skills needed to carry out the procedure efficiently, safely, and with the utmost respect for patient comfort and dignity. Let's begin our journey into the heart of phlebotomy practice.

Venipuncture is a multistep process that requires preparation, execution, and post-procedure care. Here's a step-by-step guide:
1. **Preparation:** The first step is to review the patient's information and the test orders to ensure you have the right patient and the right test. Prepare all necessary equipment, including a suitable needle, holder, blood collection tubes, gauze, tape, and alcohol wipes.
2. **Patient Identification and Verification:** Properly identify the patient using two identifiers such as the patient's name and date of birth. Check these against the information on the test order form.
3. **Patient Communication:** Inform the patient about the procedure and answer any questions they might have. Obtain the patient's consent for the procedure.

4. **Hand Hygiene and Gloves:** Perform hand hygiene and put on a new pair of gloves before starting the procedure.
5. **Site Selection:** Choose the most appropriate site for blood collection, typically a prominent vein in the antecubital area of the arm. It should be free of scars, bruises, or any signs of infection.
6. **Site Preparation:** Cleanse the area with an antiseptic wipe in a circular motion, starting from the center and moving outward.
7. **Tourniquet Application:** Apply a tourniquet about 3 to 4 inches above the venipuncture site. The tourniquet should be tight enough to cause vein distention but not so tight as to cause discomfort or halt arterial blood flow.
8. **Venipuncture:** Uncap the needle, inspect it, and perform the venipuncture with a swift, firm motion. Insert the needle at a 15 to 30-degree angle into the vein.
9. **Blood Collection:** Insert the first blood collection tube into the holder. The vacuum in the tube will draw the blood into it. If multiple tubes are required, fill them in the correct order to avoid cross-contamination of additives between tubes.
10. **Needle Withdrawal:** After the last tube is filled, release the tourniquet. Remove the needle with a swift backward motion, and immediately press down on the venipuncture site with gauze.
11. **Post-Procedural Care:** Apply a bandage to the site and ensure the patient is feeling okay before they leave. Thank them for their cooperation.
12. **Sample Labeling:** Label the tubes with the patient's information, date, and time of collection.
13. **Safe Disposal:** Safely dispose of the used needle and other sharps in a sharps container.

Remember, this is a high-level overview. Each step involves specific skills and attention to detail to ensure safety and accuracy in the procedure. It's essential for phlebotomists to be well trained and comfortable with this process.

Venipuncture can lead to several complications, and recognizing and managing them is a crucial part of a phlebotomist's role. Here are some common issues and how to handle them:
1. **Hematoma:** This occurs when blood accumulates in the tissue surrounding the vein, usually caused by the needle going through the vein or the tourniquet being left on too long. If a hematoma starts to form during the draw, immediately release the tourniquet, remove the needle, and apply firm pressure to the site.
2. **Multiple Punctures:** Sometimes, it may be challenging to locate a vein, leading to multiple attempts. If you can't find a vein after two tries, ask a colleague for assistance. This practice minimizes discomfort and potential injury to the patient.
3. **Fainting:** Some patients may faint or feel dizzy during or after the procedure. If this happens, stop the collection, lay the patient down, and ensure they are safe and monitored until they recover.
4. **Infection:** Inadequate site disinfection can lead to infection. Always clean the site thoroughly and never re-use needles. If signs of infection appear (redness, warmth, pus), advise the patient to see their doctor.

5. **Arterial Puncture:** If a pulsating flow of bright red blood is observed, you may have hit an artery instead of a vein. Stop the collection immediately, remove the needle, and apply firm pressure to the site for at least 5 minutes.
6. **Nerve Damage:** If a patient complains about sharp, shooting pain, a nerve may have been touched. Immediately withdraw the needle and select a different site for the draw.

Training and experience help phlebotomists to anticipate, prevent, and manage these and other complications. Good patient communication is also key - ensuring they know what to expect can often prevent issues from arising and helps them feel more comfortable throughout the procedure.

Unsuccessful venipuncture attempts can occur for a variety of reasons. It's crucial for a phlebotomist to manage these situations appropriately to ensure patient safety and comfort. Here are some steps to follow:
1. **Maintain a Calm Demeanor:** Keep calm and reassure the patient. Your composure can help to put the patient at ease and instill confidence.
2. **Assess the Situation:** Determine the reason for the unsuccessful attempt. It could be due to the patient's veins being too small, rolling, or deep, or due to a lack of proper hydration.
3. **Apply Pressure to the Site:** If you need to withdraw the needle without collecting blood, make sure to apply pressure to the site to prevent a hematoma.
4. **Consider Alternatives:** If you have difficulty finding a suitable vein in the antecubital area, consider other locations like the back of the hand or the wrist. However, these locations are more sensitive and should be used as secondary choices.
5. **Ask for Assistance:** If another attempt is required, it might be best to have a more experienced phlebotomist or a supervisor make the attempt, particularly if the patient is becoming distressed.
6. **Document the Attempt:** Record the unsuccessful venipuncture attempt in the patient's chart, including your observations and any patient comments.
7. **Educate the Patient:** If hydration was an issue, explain to the patient the importance of being well-hydrated before future draws. A well-hydrated vein is plumper and easier to access.

Remember, the patient's safety and comfort should always be the priority. It's better to stop an unsuccessful attempt rather than risk further discomfort or potential harm to the patient.

Capillary puncture, also known as fingerstick or heelstick (in infants), is a method of blood collection that differs substantially from venipuncture. Rather than accessing a vein, a capillary puncture collects blood from the network of tiny blood vessels (capillaries) that lies just beneath the skin surface.

The steps in capillary puncture are as follows:
1. **Choose the Site:** The site selection is often the side of the fingertip, avoiding the center of the finger pad or any callused, damaged, or diseased areas. In neonates, the outer surface of the heel is usually the best choice.

2. **Prepare the Site:** Clean the site with alcohol and allow it to air dry.
3. **Puncture the Skin:** A lancet is used to create a small puncture in the skin.
4. **Collect the Blood:** Allow a small bead of blood to form, then collect the blood with a capillary tube or onto a blood slide or reagent strip. Avoid "milking" the finger or heel, as this can dilute the sample with tissue fluid and potentially impact test results.

Capillary puncture is typically used in situations where a small volume of blood is sufficient for testing, where venous access is difficult, or where minimal invasiveness is desirable. Examples include pediatric patients, elderly patients with fragile veins, patients with needle phobia, or when only a small amount of blood is required for testing, such as glucose monitoring or hemoglobin tests.

While capillary puncture is less invasive than venipuncture, it's crucial to remember that it's still a painful procedure, especially for repeated tests like blood glucose monitoring. Proper technique, patient education, and communication are essential for ensuring patient comfort and cooperation.

Capillary puncture, sometimes known as a 'fingerstick' or 'heelstick' for neonates, is a common procedure for obtaining a small blood sample. Here is a step-by-step guide on how to perform a capillary puncture.

1. **Gather Your Equipment:** You'll need gloves, a lancet (a small, sharp instrument used to make a quick, shallow cut in the skin), an alcohol pad or swab for cleaning the site, a gauze pad or cotton ball for applying pressure after the puncture, a bandage, and capillary tubes or blood collection device designed for capillary samples.
2. **Prepare the Patient:** Just like in venipuncture, start by explaining the procedure to the patient, obtain consent if necessary, and verify their identity. Have them comfortably seated and ensure they're relaxed.
3. **Select and Clean the Site:** In adults and older children, the sides of the end of a fingertip are usually chosen. For infants, the heel is used. Avoid any areas that appear to be bruised or swollen. Clean the site with an alcohol swab and let it air dry.
4. **Perform the Puncture:** Put on your gloves. Hold the patient's finger or heel firmly. Position the lancet against the site, then trigger it to puncture the skin.
5. **Collect the Sample:** Allow a drop of blood to well up at the puncture site, then touch the collection device to the blood drop. The device should fill by capillary action. If you're using a capillary tube, be careful not to press it against the skin as it can collapse the blood drop and prevent proper filling.
6. **Apply Pressure to the Site:** Once you've collected the sample, use a clean gauze pad or cotton ball to apply pressure to the puncture site. Ask the patient to hold the gauze in place, if they're able.
7. **Seal and Label the Sample:** If you're using a capillary tube, seal the end using the specific method required for the tube type. Label the sample with the patient's information and the date and time of collection.
8. **Dispose of the Lancet and Other Waste:** Discard the lancet in a sharps container. Any other waste should be disposed of according to your facility's protocols.

9. **Provide Aftercare:** Give the patient a bandage if needed and provide any necessary aftercare instructions.

Remember, the key to a successful capillary puncture is to be gentle but firm. The procedure can be painful, but a confident, soothing demeanor can help put the patient at ease. Ensure you handle the samples properly to provide accurate and reliable test results.

During a capillary puncture, certain complications may arise. As a phlebotomist, managing these situations requires a mix of preparedness, knowledge, and skill. Here are some complications that can occur, along with how to manage them and preventative measures:

1. **Excessive Bleeding:** Applying firm pressure using a clean gauze or cotton ball on the puncture site should stop the bleeding. If the bleeding persists, continue applying pressure and seek further medical assistance. To prevent this, ensure that you've selected the correct puncture site and use the appropriate size lancet for the patient's age and physical condition.

2. **Inadequate Blood Flow:** If the blood isn't flowing sufficiently, you may need to gently massage the area from base to tip to encourage circulation. Never squeeze the site as this can cause hemolysis (breaking of the blood cells). Ensuring the patient's hand is warm before the procedure can improve circulation and prevent this issue.

3. **Pain:** The capillary puncture can be painful for some people. Using a smaller lancet can reduce pain, as can puncturing the side of the fingertip instead of the pad. A quick, assured puncture is usually less painful than a slow one.

4. **Infection:** Always clean the site thoroughly with an antiseptic before performing the puncture and apply a bandage afterward. Always wear gloves and follow your facility's protocol for infection control.

5. **Hematoma:** This can happen if blood accumulates under the skin after the puncture. Apply pressure to the site after collection to minimize this risk.

6. **Syncope (Fainting):** Some people may feel faint or dizzy during or after the procedure. If the patient starts feeling faint, have them lie down, if possible, and elevate their feet. Monitor them closely until they recover.

7. **Contamination of the Sample:** Contamination can alter test results. To prevent this, ensure the puncture site is fully dry after cleaning with the antiseptic and avoid touching the puncture site or inside of the capillary tube or specimen container.

Being aware of potential complications and prepared to manage them can help ensure the safety and comfort of the patient during a capillary puncture procedure. Good technique, careful attention to the patient, and following your facility's procedures are key.

Aftercare following venipuncture or capillary puncture is crucial to ensure a patient's comfort and to monitor for potential complications. Here are the steps to follow:

1. **Pressure Application:** Once the needle is removed from the vein, immediately apply gentle but firm pressure using a clean cotton ball or gauze on the puncture site. This assists in the coagulation process, prevents hematoma, and minimizes discomfort.

2. **Bandage Application:** After the bleeding has stopped, which usually takes a couple of minutes, apply a small adhesive bandage or dressing. This protects the wound and minimizes the risk of infection.
3. **Monitoring:** Watch the patient for a few minutes to ensure they are feeling well. Some patients may experience light-headedness or even fainting spells after a blood draw, particularly if it's their first time or they are prone to such reactions. Having them sit quietly for a while helps in recovery.
4. **Instructions:** Provide the patient with care instructions. Inform them to keep the bandage on for a few hours, avoid strenuous activity with that arm, and to monitor the site for any signs of infection or excessive bruising.
5. **Addressing Concerns:** Encourage the patient to contact the healthcare provider if they experience prolonged bleeding, excessive pain, or symptoms such as warmth, redness, and swelling at the puncture site, as these could be signs of an infection.
6. **Documentation:** After the patient leaves, document any complications or issues that occurred during the procedure, along with how these were handled.
7. **Patient Comfort:** Throughout the process, maintain a calm, reassuring demeanor to ease the patient's concerns. A positive patient experience often depends on the phlebotomist's professionalism, empathy, and communication skills.

Remember, the key to quality aftercare is monitoring the patient, clear communication, and meticulous documentation. This helps to ensure a successful procedure, promotes healing, and minimizes potential complications.

The appropriate disposal of used phlebotomy equipment is absolutely essential to the safety and hygiene of the procedure. Used needles, lancets, blood collection tubes, and other materials can present numerous risks if not disposed of correctly.

These risks primarily revolve around the potential for infection and injury. Used needles and lancets can still carry a patient's blood and any potential pathogens it might contain. If these materials are not disposed of safely, they can lead to needlestick injuries, which can transmit bloodborne pathogens such as hepatitis B, hepatitis C, or HIV.

Further, improper disposal can cause environmental pollution. If sharp wastes find their way into regular trash, they could harm sanitation workers, end up in landfills, or contribute to pollution if they are incinerated under unsuitable conditions.

To mitigate these risks, all used phlebotomy equipment should be disposed of in designated sharps containers. These are puncture-resistant containers that are typically color-coded and labeled to indicate that they contain biohazardous materials. The containers should be located as close as possible to the point of use.

Also, phlebotomists should never attempt to recap needles, which can lead to accidental sticks. In addition, full sharps containers should be replaced promptly to prevent overfilling, which can also increase the risk of injury.

Lastly, all healthcare facilities should comply with local, state, and national regulations for the final disposal of biohazardous waste. This often involves engaging the services of a licensed medical waste disposal company, which can ensure that the waste is treated and disposed of in a safe, compliant manner.

Handling blood specimens post-collection is a critical process that can significantly influence the quality of the samples, and in turn, the accuracy of laboratory results. Here are some general guidelines for proper storage and handling of blood samples.

1. Labeling: Immediately after collection, each blood sample should be correctly labeled. The label typically includes the patient's name, date and time of collection, and identifier like a patient ID number or barcode. It's essential never to pre-label tubes before collection, and always double-check the information with the patient.
2. Mixing: If you've collected blood into tubes with additives (like anticoagulants), gently invert the tubes several times to mix the blood with the additive. This prevents clotting in the anticoagulant tubes and ensures homogeneous mixing in tubes with other additives. Avoid vigorous shaking, as this could lead to hemolysis - rupture of the red blood cells, which can interfere with many tests.
3. Transport: Blood samples should be transported to the laboratory as quickly as possible. If there's a delay, make sure you store them properly. Tubes should be transported in upright position to prevent spillage or leakage.
4. Storage: The storage conditions will depend on the type of test ordered. Many blood tests require the samples to be stored and transported at room temperature (15-25°C). Some may require refrigeration (2-8°C), especially if the test isn't going to be performed right away. Rarely, samples may need to be frozen (-20°C or lower). The lab should provide guidance on proper storage conditions.
5. Time Sensitivity: Certain blood tests are time-sensitive. For instance, glucose levels in a blood sample can decrease if not processed within a couple of hours. Again, communication with the lab is crucial to understanding the stability of the analyte of interest.
6. Integrity: Don't use damaged or leaking tubes. If a tube is compromised, it can affect the specimen quality and even pose a biohazard risk.

By observing these steps, phlebotomists can ensure that they handle, store, and transport blood samples in a manner that preserves their integrity, leading to accurate and reliable lab results.

Managing and reporting adverse events or complications after venipuncture or capillary puncture is crucial for patient safety and for continuous improvement of healthcare procedures. Here's a general outline of the process:

1. Assessment and Immediate Action: In the event of an adverse reaction or complication, the first step is to ensure the patient's well-being. Stop the procedure, if necessary, and provide appropriate immediate care based on the situation, like applying pressure to a site that's bleeding excessively.
2. Documentation: Document the event as soon as possible, while the details are still fresh. The information should include the patient's identification details, the date and time of the event, a detailed description of the event and any signs or symptoms, steps taken in response, and the patient's condition after those steps. The documentation should also include information about the procedure, like the site of puncture and the method used. It's crucial to remain factual and objective in the documentation.
3. Reporting: Inform a supervisor or a designated person within your organization about the incident. In many settings, there's a formal incident report form to be completed. Some serious adverse events might also need to be reported to external organizations, like a health department or a regulatory body - follow your facility's policy about this.
4. Follow-up: The patient might need additional care, like a follow-up appointment or a referral to another healthcare provider. Make sure this is arranged and that the patient understands the plan.
5. Review and Learning: Ideally, each adverse event should lead to a review of procedures, with the goal of preventing similar incidents in the future. You might participate in this process, for example, by providing additional details about the event, or by contributing to a discussion about ways to improve procedures.

Remember, the specifics of the reporting procedure might vary depending on your location and the policies of your healthcare facility. It's essential to familiarize yourself with these policies so you can respond appropriately if an adverse event occurs.

Section 4: Special Collections and Point of Care Testing:

As we delve into the fourth section of our guide, we turn our attention towards more specialized procedures within the realm of phlebotomy. This section, titled 'Special Collections and Point of Care Testing', expands our study to encompass areas such as collection of blood cultures, arterial blood gases, and the administration of glucose tolerance tests, among other specialized collections.

In addition, we explore the increasingly significant area of Point of Care Testing (POCT). POCT refers to medical diagnostic tests performed outside the traditional laboratory setting, typically at the bedside or near the patient. These tests, while smaller in scale, provide rapid results and can play a crucial role in patient care. This section discusses common types of POCT, procedures, and the responsibilities and considerations a phlebotomist must understand to execute these tests effectively.

The primary objective of this section is to enhance your understanding of these special collections and tests, ensuring that you're equipped with the necessary knowledge and competence to handle these tasks in a professional healthcare setting. As with the previous sections, we'll ensure the information is detailed, comprehensive, and presented in an easy-to-understand manner, setting you up for success in your phlebotomy career.

Blood culture collections are a critical component of diagnostic procedures in healthcare, especially when it comes to identifying infections that are present in the bloodstream, commonly referred to as bacteremia or septicemia. These collections are vital for determining the type of organism causing the infection, which helps clinicians decide the most effective course of treatment.

Unlike standard venipuncture, blood culture collections require specific collection and handling procedures. The goal is to maximize the detection of pathogenic organisms while minimizing the risk of contamination that could lead to false-positive results.

In standard venipuncture, blood is drawn directly into a tube for further testing. However, in a blood culture collection, the blood is injected into bottles containing a nutrient broth. These bottles provide an environment that promotes the growth of bacteria and fungi, making it easier to detect an infection.

Another difference lies in the volume of blood collected. Blood cultures typically require larger volumes of blood since the likelihood of detecting microorganisms increases with the blood volume. This differs from standard venipuncture where the volume is often smaller and defined by the specific test required.

Additionally, sterility is of utmost importance in blood culture collections. The skin must be thoroughly disinfected to avoid introducing skin flora into the culture bottles, which could result in false positives. The bottle tops must also be disinfected before blood inoculation.

Lastly, blood cultures are often drawn from two different sites or at two different times to increase the chance of detecting intermittent bacteremia and to differentiate between true pathogens and contaminants. Standard venipuncture, on the other hand, is usually a one-time event.

Collecting a blood culture is a meticulous process that needs to be performed with great care to ensure the integrity of the sample and prevent contamination. Here are the step-by-step instructions:

1. **Prepare Your Equipment:** Gather all necessary equipment, including blood culture bottles (aerobic and anaerobic), a tourniquet, needles, syringes, alcohol wipes, chlorhexidine, and sterile gloves. The patient's skin, the culture bottles, and the phlebotomist's hands should all be thoroughly cleaned to prevent contamination.
2. **Identify the Patient:** Ask the patient to state their full name and date of birth. Compare this information with the details on the requisition form and the patient's wristband to ensure correct patient identification.
3. **Position the Patient:** The patient should be comfortable, with their arm in a relaxed, extended position.
4. **Select and Prepare the Venipuncture Site:** Apply the tourniquet and assess for a suitable vein. Once the vein has been identified, release the tourniquet temporarily. Cleanse the venipuncture site starting at the center and working outward in a circular motion using chlorhexidine. Allow it to dry completely before proceeding.
5. **Perform the Venipuncture:** Put on sterile gloves and reapply the tourniquet. With a sterile needle and syringe, perform the venipuncture.
6. **Collect the Blood:** Once blood flow is established, fill the syringe with the appropriate volume of blood. Most blood culture bottles will indicate the volume of blood needed for an optimal yield.
7. **Inoculate the Blood Culture Bottles:** Release the tourniquet. Disinfect the tops of the blood culture bottles with alcohol before inoculating the blood. Inoculate the aerobic bottle first, then the anaerobic bottle.
8. **End the Venipuncture:** After the blood has been inoculated into the bottles, remove the needle from the patient's arm using a swift backward motion. Apply gentle pressure to the site with a gauze pad.
9. **Label the Specimens and Document:** Label the blood culture bottles with the patient's information and the time of collection. Document the procedure in the patient's medical record, including any observations about the procedure.

Remember, the main precaution during this procedure is to maintain sterility to prevent contamination. Any breach of aseptic technique can lead to false-positive results, potentially leading to unnecessary treatments for the patient. Every step must be performed with care and attention to detail.

A glucose tolerance test (GTT) is commonly indicated for diagnosing conditions related to glucose metabolism, such as diabetes mellitus, gestational diabetes, insulin resistance, or reactive hypoglycemia. Its main purpose is to check how well the body handles glucose after consumption.

The administration of a GTT usually follows these steps:

1. **Patient Preparation:** The patient is instructed to maintain their regular diet and exercise pattern for at least three days before the test. Additionally, they are asked to fast for 8-12 hours before the test. It's crucial that the patient understands and adheres to these instructions, as their actions may influence the test results.

2. **Fasting Blood Sample Collection:** The phlebotomist first collects a blood sample to measure the fasting blood glucose level. This serves as the baseline measurement.

3. **Glucose Administration:** The patient is given a glucose solution to drink. For adults, the standard dose is usually 75 grams of glucose dissolved in water. For pregnant women being screened for gestational diabetes, the dose is typically 50 grams.

4. **Subsequent Blood Samples:** Additional blood samples are taken at timed intervals after the glucose solution is consumed, commonly at one, two, and sometimes three hours. These samples allow the healthcare provider to see how the patient's body is processing the glucose over time.

5. **Interpretation of Results:** A healthcare provider will interpret the results. If the blood glucose levels are higher than normal at any of the testing times, it could suggest a problem with the body's ability to process glucose, indicating a condition like diabetes.

Remember, the GTT is a prolonged procedure that requires patient compliance and careful timing. Mistakes in timing can significantly impact the results, leading to inaccurate diagnosis and treatment.

Carrying out a glucose tolerance test (GTT) requires careful preparation and methodical steps to ensure valid results. Here's a detailed guide:

1. **Pre-Test Instructions:** Inform the patient about the procedure well in advance. Explain that they will need to fast for 8-12 hours prior to the test, but they should continue their normal diet and exercise routine in the days leading up to the test. Also, advise the patient to avoid smoking, alcohol, and caffeine on the day of the test.

2. **Patient Verification:** Confirm the patient's identity according to your lab's protocol. Ensure the patient has followed the pre-test instructions correctly, especially the fasting requirement.

3. **Initial Blood Sample:** The first step in the actual procedure is to collect a fasting blood sample. This sample will provide the baseline glucose level.

4. **Glucose Consumption:** Next, provide the patient with a glucose solution to drink. The standard dose for adults is 75 grams of glucose, while pregnant women being screened for gestational diabetes typically receive 50 grams.

5. **Timed Blood Samples:** Collect blood samples at specific intervals after the patient consumes the glucose solution. The usual practice is to draw samples at one hour, two hours, and possibly three hours. Make sure to stick to the exact timing for each draw as this is crucial for the validity of the test.
6. **Patient Comfort:** Ensure the patient is comfortable throughout the procedure as it can be quite lengthy. They should remain seated and refrain from physical activity during the test to avoid affecting the results.
7. **Data Recording:** Label each sample with the patient's information and the time of collection. Record any relevant patient information, such as symptoms experienced during the test.
8. **Post-Test Care:** Once all samples are collected, apply pressure to the puncture site until bleeding stops. Provide aftercare instructions, which generally include resuming normal diet and activities.
9. **Sample Storage and Transportation:** Store and transport the samples properly to the lab for analysis. Each lab may have specific requirements for this step.

Remember, accuracy in timing and sample handling are critical in GTT to avoid any erroneous results. If the patient feels unwell at any point during the test, especially if symptoms of hypoglycemia like dizziness, sweating, or feeling faint occur, immediate care should be provided.

Therapeutic phlebotomy is a medical procedure that involves removing a certain volume of blood from a patient's body as part of the treatment for specific medical conditions. Its primary purpose is to reduce the amount of excess iron or red blood cells in the bloodstream.

Here are some conditions where therapeutic phlebotomy is typically indicated:
1. **Polycythemia Vera:** This is a slow-growing blood cancer where your bone marrow makes too many red blood cells, leading to a thickening of the blood which can cause clots. Therapeutic phlebotomy is used to reduce the concentration of red blood cells.
2. **Hemochromatosis:** This is an iron disorder in which the body simply loads too much iron. This excess iron is stored in body tissues and organs, particularly the skin, heart, liver, pancreas, and joints. Regular therapeutic phlebotomy helps remove the excess iron from the body.
3. **Porphyria Cutanea Tarda:** This is the most common type of porphyria, where the body lacks an enzyme needed to balance the production of heme, a component of hemoglobin. Therapeutic phlebotomy is used to reduce heme levels.

These are just a few examples. The procedure itself is similar to donating blood, but the frequency and volume of removal would be specific to the patient's condition and doctor's instructions. It's crucial to monitor patients for symptoms of anemia or other side effects, given that the procedure involves removing significant amounts of blood. Regular lab tests are also needed to ensure the effectiveness of the treatment.

Therapeutic phlebotomy is carried out much like a regular blood donation, but it's crucial to follow the specific guidelines set out by the treating physician, given the medical purpose behind the procedure. Here's a basic outline of the steps involved:

1. **Assessment:** Assess the patient's health status and review their medical history. Check the physician's order for specific instructions regarding volume of blood to be removed and frequency of procedures.
2. **Informed Consent:** Before the procedure, ensure the patient understands why the therapeutic phlebotomy is necessary and what it entails. Obtain informed consent.
3. **Preparation:** Have the patient sit comfortably. Apply a tourniquet to the upper arm to make the veins more visible.
4. **Vein Selection and Puncture:** Select an appropriate vein, ideally in the antecubital space where veins are larger and closer to the surface. Cleanse the area thoroughly with an antiseptic to minimize risk of infection, and then perform the venipuncture.
5. **Blood Draw:** Draw the blood slowly into a blood bag, monitoring the patient throughout. The volume of blood removed will depend on the physician's order but typically ranges from 250-500 ml.
6. **Ending the Procedure:** Once the required amount of blood has been drawn, remove the needle and apply pressure to the site with a gauze pad to stop bleeding. Afterward, apply a bandage.
7. **Post-Procedure Care:** Monitor the patient for a short while to ensure they don't show signs of dizziness or fainting. Encourage them to have a snack and hydrate.

There are several precautions that need to be taken during therapeutic phlebotomy:

- **Monitoring the Patient:** The patient should be monitored continuously for any adverse reactions, such as dizziness, fainting, or feeling unwell. If these occur, the procedure should be stopped immediately.
- **Maintaining Sterility:** Sterility should be maintained throughout the procedure to prevent infection.
- **Volume Control:** It's essential to avoid removing too much blood, which could potentially lead to anemia. The volume to be removed should be as per the physician's instruction.

The potential complications that could arise from therapeutic phlebotomy include anemia, infection at the puncture site, fainting or dizziness due to sudden decrease in blood volume, and in rare cases, iron deficiency if the procedure is performed too frequently. As always, it's important to have clear communication with the patient about possible signs of complications and when to seek medical attention.

Point of Care Testing (POCT) refers to medical testing that is performed at or near the location of the patient. The term encapsulates any analytical test administered outside the conventional laboratory setting, typically at the patient's bedside or in close proximity.

POCT's value in modern healthcare is multifold:

Timely Results: One of the key advantages of POCT is the speed of obtaining results. By reducing the turnaround time associated with sending samples to a laboratory and waiting for results, healthcare providers can make quicker diagnoses and decisions about treatment, enhancing patient care.

Improved Patient Experience: POCT allows for more interactive, personalized care, as the patient is involved in the testing process. This can lead to increased patient satisfaction and better engagement in their own healthcare.

Convenience: With POCT, a broad range of tests can be performed in a variety of settings such as home, ambulance, surgery centers, or rural areas, without the need for a full-scale laboratory. This makes healthcare more accessible, especially for those who may find it difficult to access traditional lab services.

Cost Efficiency: By delivering results faster, POCT may reduce hospital admission rates, lengths of hospital stays, and overall healthcare costs.

Precision Medicine: POCT also plays a significant role in the delivery of precision medicine, where treatments are tailored to individual patients. Rapid tests can provide immediate information about a patient's genetic makeup or specific disease markers, enabling customized treatment.

In summary, POCT has revolutionized the way we approach diagnostics by making it more patient-centered, efficient, and in many cases, cost-effective. As technology continues to advance, the role of POCT in healthcare is likely to grow further.

Benefits of Point of Care Testing (POCT) compared to traditional laboratory testing include:
1. **Faster Results:** POCT can deliver results within minutes, as opposed to hours or days with traditional lab testing. This immediate feedback allows for quicker decision making, which can be critical in emergency situations.
2. **Improved Patient Care:** By providing immediate results, POCT allows for more efficient patient management. Treatment can be initiated sooner, which can lead to improved patient outcomes.
3. **Convenience:** POCT can be performed at the patient's bedside or in the community, making it more accessible to those who have difficulty accessing traditional lab services. This can reduce the time and cost associated with traveling to and from labs for both patients and healthcare providers.
4. **Increased Patient Engagement:** POCT often involves the patient in the testing process, fostering a more interactive and personalized healthcare experience. This can increase patient satisfaction and engagement in their own healthcare.
However, there are also challenges associated with POCT:
1. **Quality Control:** POCT devices are subject to environmental conditions such as temperature and humidity, which can affect results. In addition, as these tests are often performed by non-

laboratory personnel, there may be greater variation in how the tests are conducted, which can impact accuracy and reliability.

2. Cost: The per-test cost of POCT can be higher than traditional lab testing. Although it may lead to overall cost savings by reducing hospital stays or preventing complications, the upfront cost may be a barrier for some institutions or patients.

3. Regulatory Compliance: POCT is subject to regulation, and all tests must meet the same regulatory requirements as traditional lab tests. Meeting these requirements can be challenging, especially for smaller healthcare facilities or those without dedicated laboratory personnel.

4. Limited Test Menu: While the range of available POCT is expanding, it still cannot match the extensive testing capabilities of a traditional lab. Complex tests that require sophisticated equipment are generally not available as POCT.

In conclusion, while POCT offers many advantages over traditional laboratory testing, careful consideration must be given to the challenges it presents to ensure accurate, reliable testing.

A phlebotomist's role in Point of Care Testing (POCT) can be quite diverse and comes with several responsibilities. Here's what the role typically involves:

1. Test Administration: The phlebotomist is often responsible for administering the test. This includes preparing the patient, collecting the specimen (usually through a fingerstick or sometimes a venipuncture), applying the sample to the test device, and conducting the test following the manufacturer's instructions.

2. Equipment Maintenance: Phlebotomists are responsible for ensuring that testing equipment is in good working order. This includes routine cleaning and maintenance tasks, as well as troubleshooting any problems that might arise.

3. Quality Control: Phlebotomists must perform regular quality control checks to ensure the test is working correctly and providing accurate results. This might involve running control samples or completing checks of the device.

4. Record Keeping: It is crucial to keep accurate records of each test conducted, including the test results, date and time of the test, any issues or anomalies observed, and other relevant details.

5. Patient Interaction: Phlebotomists are often the point of contact for the patient, so they need to be able to explain the procedure, answer any questions, and sometimes even relay the test results. This requires good communication skills and a sensitivity to the patient's needs and concerns.

6. Compliance with Protocols: Lastly, it's crucial that phlebotomists follow the established protocols for the specific POCT being performed. This includes not only the testing procedure itself, but also infection control measures, safety protocols, and confidentiality requirements.

In terms of additional skills, phlebotomists involved in POCT need a firm understanding of the tests they're performing and the equipment they're using. They need to be detail-oriented to ensure the tests are conducted correctly and the results are accurate. They also need strong problem-solving skills, as they may need to troubleshoot issues with the testing equipment. Furthermore, good communication skills are essential for effectively interacting with patients and other healthcare professionals.

Let's delve into two common Point of Care Tests (POCTs): glucose monitoring and coagulation testing. Both of these tests are essential tools in managing chronic diseases and have specific procedures and equipment needed to ensure accurate results.

1. Glucose Monitoring:

Glucose monitoring is used to measure the amount of sugar, or glucose, in a patient's blood. It's frequently used by people with diabetes to monitor their blood sugar levels.

Equipment Needed:

- Glucose meter: This device measures the glucose concentration.
- Test strips: These are specially designed strips for the specific glucose meter being used.
- Lancets: These are small, sharp objects used to prick the finger.
- Alcohol swabs: For cleaning the area before the finger prick.

Procedure:

- Begin by washing your hands and putting on gloves.
- Clean the patient's finger with an alcohol swab and let it air dry.
- Use the lancet to prick the side of the patient's finger.
- Wipe away the first drop of blood with a clean gauze pad.
- Squeeze the finger gently to obtain a new drop of blood.
- Touch the edge of the test strip to the blood drop, allowing the blood to be drawn into the strip.
- Insert the test strip into the meter and wait for the results.
- Dispose of used materials properly.

2. Coagulation Testing:

Coagulation testing, specifically the Prothrombin Time/International Normalized Ratio (PT/INR) test, is a blood test that measures the time it takes for your blood to clot. It's often performed on patients taking anticoagulant medications.

Equipment Needed:

- Coagulation meter: This device measures the clotting ability of the blood.
- PT/INR test strips or cartridges: These contain chemicals that initiate the clotting process in the blood sample.
- Lancets: For pricking the finger.
- Alcohol swabs: For cleaning the area before the finger prick.

Procedure:

- As with glucose testing, start by washing your hands and donning gloves.
- Clean the patient's finger with an alcohol swab and let it air dry.

- Prick the patient's finger with the lancet.
- Wipe away the first drop of blood.
- Collect the next drop of blood onto the test strip or into the cartridge (depending on your device).
- Insert the test strip or cartridge into the meter and wait for the results.
- Dispose of used materials properly.

In both cases, it's essential to follow the manufacturer's instructions for the specific devices and test materials you're using. Remember, patient comfort and safety are paramount throughout these procedures.

Quality control measures in Point of Care Testing (POCT) are integral for ensuring the accuracy and reliability of test results. It's all about maintaining confidence in your data and providing the best possible patient care.

1. Use of Control Materials:
Control materials are substances that contain a known amount of the analyte being measured. They should be tested routinely, following the manufacturer's instructions. These materials behave similarly to patient samples and provide a benchmark to compare the patient's results. If the control material results are within the expected range, you can have confidence in the accuracy of the patient's results.

2. Regular Device Maintenance:
Like any piece of medical equipment, POCT devices require regular maintenance to ensure their proper functioning. This may include cleaning, calibration, and other manufacturer-recommended actions. Regular maintenance helps prevent unexpected device malfunctions that could affect the test results.

3. Staff Training:
The person performing the POCT, often a phlebotomist, should be adequately trained and competent. They should understand the procedure, know how to use the device correctly, and be aware of potential sources of error. Refreshing training periodically is also a good practice to ensure ongoing competency.

4. Follow Manufacturer's Instructions:
The device manufacturer's instructions should be followed rigorously. This includes how to perform the test, how to handle and store test strips or cartridges, how to maintain the device, and what to do if control material results are out of range.

5. Record Keeping:

Document everything - patient results, control results, device maintenance, and any troubleshooting or actions taken if the control results were out of range. Proper record keeping is crucial for traceability and can provide valuable information if a problem arises.

6. Participate in External Quality Assurance (EQA) Programs:
EQA programs involve testing samples provided by an external organization and comparing your results with laboratories or POCT sites elsewhere. Participation in these programs provides an additional layer of assurance in your testing quality.

By incorporating these quality control measures into their routine, phlebotomists play an essential role in ensuring the accuracy and reliability of POCT results.

Documenting and reporting Point of Care Testing (POCT) results are critical steps in the testing process, having direct implications for patient care. As POCTs are often used in critical care situations where immediate clinical decisions need to be made, the precise documentation and prompt reporting of these results can significantly impact patient outcomes.

Here are the key steps involved in documenting and reporting POCT results:

1. Documenting the Test Results:
Every test result should be accurately documented at the time the test is completed. This includes the patient's identification details, the date and time of the test, the test result, and any relevant comments, such as if the patient was fasting. Digital POCT devices often record these details automatically. However, manual recording might be needed in some situations.

2. Reporting the Test Results:
Test results need to be promptly communicated to the relevant healthcare provider, often electronically through a laboratory information system. The test result alone might not be meaningful, so it's important to report any pertinent clinical observations or patient comments that may help interpret the results.

3. Confirming Receipt:
Always ensure that the healthcare provider has received the test results, particularly if the results indicate a critical situation.

4. Follow-up Documentation:
Any actions taken based on the test results, such as medication changes, should also be documented.

Documentation of POCT results is essential for several reasons:

1. Patient Safety:

Accurate documentation ensures that healthcare providers base their decisions on correct data, reducing the risk of misdiagnosis or inappropriate treatment.

2. Legal Requirements:
Medical records, including test results, are legal documents. They can be used as evidence in legal cases related to patient care.

3. Continuity of Care:
Test results become a part of the patient's medical history, informing future medical decisions.

4. Quality Assurance:
Documented results allow for quality control and quality assurance processes, helping to maintain the reliability of the POCT procedures.

5. Research and Public Health:
Aggregated test results can be used in research studies and public health surveillance.

In summary, thorough documentation and accurate reporting of POCT results are vital to delivering safe and effective patient care, meeting legal requirements, ensuring continuity of care, maintaining testing quality, and contributing to research and public health efforts.

Phlebotomists play an integral role in the utilization and development of Point of Care Testing (POCT) within their practice. By continually striving for improvement and optimization, phlebotomists can contribute to the overall effectiveness of POCT. Here are some ways they can make a difference:

1. Continuing Education:
Phlebotomists should stay informed about the latest developments in POCT technology and methodologies. This knowledge can enhance their skills and allow them to use POCT devices more effectively. Educational seminars, workshops, and online courses can be beneficial sources of such knowledge.

2. Advocating for Quality Control:
Phlebotomists can actively participate in implementing and promoting quality control measures in POCT. This could include regularly maintaining and calibrating equipment, accurately documenting test results, and participating in internal and external quality assurance programs.

3. Patient Education:
Phlebotomists often serve as the bridge between patients and laboratory services. They can educate patients about the POCT process, explaining the purpose of the tests, the meaning of results, and the importance of accurate specimen collection.

4. Interprofessional Collaboration:
Working closely with other healthcare professionals can enhance the overall effectiveness of POCT. By sharing insights about the practical aspects of POCT and offering suggestions based on frontline experiences, phlebotomists can contribute to the development of more effective protocols and procedures.

5. Feedback and Innovation:
Given their hands-on experience, phlebotomists can provide valuable feedback about POCT devices and procedures. They can suggest improvements to enhance efficiency, accuracy, or user-friendliness. This feedback can drive innovation and optimization in POCT technology and methodology.

6. Compliance with Regulations:
Phlebotomists should be well-versed with all the local, state, and national regulations governing POCT. Adherence to these regulations not only ensures the legality of their practice but also contributes to the overall safety and effectiveness of POCT.

By leveraging these strategies, phlebotomists can significantly contribute to improving and optimizing POCT within their practice. Their proactive involvement in this area is critical to ensuring that POCT serves as an effective tool in enhancing patient care and health outcomes.

Section 5: Processing and Handling:

Welcome to Section 5: Processing and Handling. This section of the study guide provides a detailed overview of the critical procedures and guidelines that follow specimen collection, ensuring that these specimens are suitable for accurate analysis and diagnostics. Proper processing and handling of specimens are fundamental for maintaining their integrity, and it's a responsibility that phlebotomists share along with the rest of the laboratory team.

In this section, we will explore the necessary steps and precautions to take after blood and other specimens have been collected. We will discuss topics such as specimen transportation, centrifugation, aliquoting, and storage, as well as the importance of timely and correct data entry into the laboratory information system.

Additionally, we will delve into the rules for handling special specimens, such as those needing immediate processing or those collected for molecular diagnostics. The handling of biohazardous materials and the procedures for decontaminating and maintaining a clean and safe workspace will also be covered.

A deep understanding of these topics will not only enhance the accuracy and reliability of the test results but also contribute to efficient laboratory operations and ultimately improve patient care. This knowledge is essential for phlebotomists, given the vital role they play in the healthcare team. By the end of this section, you will have gained a comprehensive understanding of the importance of proper specimen handling and the specific steps needed to achieve this in a clinical setting. Let's dive in!

The importance of proper specimen handling in a clinical laboratory setting cannot be overstated. Let's unravel why, shall we?

At the heart of any clinical lab is the objective to provide accurate and reliable test results, as these greatly influence patient diagnosis, management, and treatment. The process begins not at the analysis stage but way earlier, with specimen collection and handling.

Maintaining the integrity of the specimen is absolutely pivotal to achieving accurate test results. From the moment a sample is collected, each step in its handling can potentially alter its composition and, in turn, the test outcomes. This involves everything from the initial collection method, labeling, storage, transportation to the lab, and eventually to the processing and analysis stages.

For example, if a blood sample isn't mixed properly with the anticoagulant in the collection tube, it can clot before analysis, leading to inaccurate results. Incorrect labeling can lead to mix-ups, causing patients to get erroneous results. Improper storage or delay in transportation can trigger chemical changes in the sample, which may skew the test readings.

In essence, diligent specimen handling is the unsung hero, ensuring that the snapshot of the patient's health status taken at the time of collection remains unaltered until it is analyzed. As such, it plays a pivotal role in maintaining the quality of test results and, by extension, in quality patient care. Let's not forget that patients make health decisions based on these results, so the onus is on us to keep this picture as pristine as possible, don't you think?

Delving into the factors that can affect the integrity of specimens after collection is like walking into a maze - it's a complex and nuanced terrain, but I promise to guide you through.

One factor that can affect a specimen's integrity is temperature. Certain samples like blood cultures should be kept at room temperature, while others, like a urine culture, require refrigeration to slow down bacterial growth. Specimens for some tests may even require freezing to halt any ongoing biochemical reactions.

Then we have the factor of time. The longer the period between sample collection and analysis, the greater the chances for biochemical changes, which can alter test results. Therefore, it is crucial to process and analyze samples as soon as possible.

Improper handling can also lead to hemolysis (rupture of red blood cells), which can cause falsely elevated results for certain tests like potassium. Care should be taken while drawing blood, handling, and transporting samples to prevent this.

Contamination is another factor to consider. This can occur at various stages, from collection to processing. For instance, contamination of a sterile urine sample can occur if the container touches non-sterile surfaces or if the patient's skin is not properly cleaned before collection.

To mitigate these factors, meticulous attention to each detail of the pre-analytical phase is paramount. This involves proper patient preparation, right choice of specimen collection devices, correct technique of specimen collection, accurate labeling, and appropriate storage conditions. Not to mention, timely transportation to the laboratory and ensuring minimal delay before processing and analysis.

Let's also emphasize the importance of adhering to the specific handling instructions for each type of test, as they may vary widely. The goal? Maintain the specimen's integrity just as it was in the patient's body, minimizing any chance of error, and ensuring the reliability of test results. It's like preserving the scene of an event, without any alteration, for the most accurate understanding of the event. That's our goal as diligent caregivers, don't you agree?

Dealing with blood specimens immediately after collection is akin to handling a delicate piece of art. It's both a science and an art, requiring precision, knowledge, and great care. Let's walk through the process together.

After collection, gently invert anticoagulated blood tubes 8-10 times. This gentle mixing action helps distribute the anticoagulant throughout the blood to prevent clotting. Be careful not to shake the tubes, as this can cause hemolysis.

Next, observe the sample for any signs of hemolysis or clotting, as these may affect the quality of the sample and thus the accuracy of the results. Also, it's a good practice to check for sufficient sample volume as some tests may require a minimum amount of sample.

The labeling of the specimen is of utmost importance and should be done immediately after collection, while still at the patient's bedside. The label should include at least the patient's full name, date of birth, date and time of collection, and the initials of the person who collected the sample. Some institutions may also require additional identifiers like patient ID number.

Remember, labeling should never be done before collection, and pre-printed labels should be cross-verified with the patient's ID band and the test requisition to ensure accuracy. Any error in labeling can lead to serious consequences, including misdiagnosis and inappropriate treatment.

After the labeling, specimens should be placed in a biohazard bag for transportation. The bag usually has two sections - the larger one for the specimens and a smaller attached pouch for the requisition form or any paperwork. Seal the bag properly to avoid any leakages or spills during transportation.

In a nutshell, handling of blood specimens after collection is an incredibly critical step that requires scrupulous attention to detail. It's the key to ensure the integrity of the samples, ensuring that the results provided to physicians paint an accurate picture of the patient's health. We, as healthcare providers, play an instrumental role in this process, don't you think?

Transporting specimens - it's not quite like delivering a pizza, is it? It involves certain guidelines to protect both the integrity of the samples and the safety of everyone involved. Let's delve into this topic!

When transporting specimens within a healthcare facility, you'll want to make sure they are secured in a leak-proof, sturdy container. This might often be a biohazard bag or a transport box. Ensure that these containers are not overfilled and have a secure lid to avoid any spillages or breakages.

Now, it's important to remember that different types of specimens might have different transportation requirements. For instance, some samples need to be refrigerated or kept on ice, while others need to be maintained at room temperature. You need to be aware of these requirements and handle the samples accordingly.

Equally crucial is to protect the paperwork. Often, the lab request form or manifest travels with the specimen. To prevent it from being soiled or lost, it's usually placed in a separate pouch or compartment.

Now, what happens when specimens need to be sent to an external lab, you ask? The process is similar, but with a few additional precautions. First, it's vital to ensure that all specimens are appropriately packaged and sealed to meet transport regulations. You would also need to use a transport carrier that complies with local and national transportation regulations.

Furthermore, the transportation box or package needs to be marked with the appropriate hazard labels. These may include biohazard symbols or other specific warnings based on the nature of the specimen.

Lastly, remember to document everything. This includes information like the date and time of dispatch, the carrier details, and the names of the people involved in the transportation. This record can help trace back any issues if they arise.

In a nutshell, whether it's a short trip down the corridor to the in-house lab or a longer journey to an external facility, transporting specimens is a crucial task that requires meticulous attention. Always stay mindful, be aware of the guidelines, and handle with care - that's our mantra!

Storage conditions for specimens—now that's an area that requires precision and understanding! It's like the climate control for precious artifacts in a museum. Every sample, like every masterpiece, has its ideal conditions for preservation.

Let's start with blood specimens, a commonly dealt with sample type in phlebotomy. The storage requirements of these specimens often depend on the type of test being performed. For instance:

1. **Serum Samples:** Once the blood has been collected and clotted, and the serum is separated by centrifugation, it's generally recommended to analyze the serum as soon as possible. If the analysis can't be performed immediately, the serum can be stored in the refrigerator (around 2 to 8 degrees Celsius) for up to 48 hours. For longer periods, freezing the serum at -20 degrees Celsius or colder would be the way to go.
2. **Plasma Samples:** Similar to serum, if immediate analysis isn't possible, you can refrigerate the plasma for a short time. For longer periods, freezing is necessary.
3. **Whole Blood:** Certain tests, such as those for complete blood counts (CBC), require whole blood. These samples are typically stored at room temperature and should be analyzed within a few hours of collection.

However, these are general guidelines. Some tests have very specific requirements. For example, samples for a potassium test should not be refrigerated, as it can cause the cells to burst, increasing the potassium levels in the serum. Likewise, samples for a blood gas analysis should be analyzed immediately and, until then, be kept at room temperature without any delays.

In addition, it's important to store specimens in a way that avoids cross-contamination, preserves the identity of the specimen, and maintains the sterility of unused containers or supplies.

Remember, proper storage not only preserves the integrity of specimens but also ensures the accuracy of test results. So, in your journey as a phlebotomist, make sure to follow the storage guidelines meticulously. It's like being a custodian for these microscopic works of art!

Getting into the nitty-gritty of handling specimens that need refrigeration or freezing, let's understand this is akin to preserving perishable foods. The right temperature can keep the specimen 'fresh'—the integrity intact—so accurate results can be derived.

1. **Timing Matters:** Once the blood has been collected, processed (if required), and separated, specimens that need refrigeration should be promptly put in the fridge. Likewise, those requiring freezing should be placed in the freezer without delay. Procrastination is a specimen's worst enemy!

2. **Correct Temperature:** Remember, the refrigerator should be between 2 to 8 degrees Celsius, and the freezer should be -20 degrees Celsius or colder. Regular checks and maintenance of this equipment are a must to ensure they are working correctly. Consider it part of your role as a lab superhero.

3. **Avoiding Freeze-Thaw Cycles:** Repeated freezing and thawing can degrade the specimen, so avoid these cycles as much as possible. Once a specimen is frozen, it should stay frozen until it's time for testing.

4. **Proper Labeling and Packaging:** Even in the cold, your specimens need their identities! Make sure they are labeled properly before being stored. This usually includes the patient's name, identification number, date, and time of collection.

5. **Don't Overstuff:** Just like you don't overstuff your refrigerator at home (Well, ideally!), the same rule applies here. Overcrowding can lead to inconsistent temperatures and potential cross-contamination.

Common mistakes? Leaving specimens at room temperature for too long before refrigeration or freezing, improper labeling, incorrect temperatures, and repeated freeze-thaw cycles. These errors can alter the specimen's integrity, leading to inaccurate test results.

The rules of handling specimens needing cold storage might seem many, but as you immerse in your role, they'll become second nature. The goal is clear—keep that specimen in the best condition for accurate results. You're like the guardian of the 'specimen universe'!

The term 'chain of custody' may make you feel like you've suddenly been thrust into a crime TV show, and, in essence, you're not entirely far off. In the context of phlebotomy and laboratory testing, 'chain of custody' refers to the documentation and procedural control of a specimen from the moment it's collected from a patient, to processing, to analysis, and even to the disposal or storing stages.

When it comes to tests with potential legal implications, like drug testing or forensic samples, the chain of custody becomes particularly critical. These tests can affect employment decisions, legal proceedings, or even criminal investigations. Therefore, it's absolutely essential that the results are accurate and that the specimen is unquestionably connected to the individual from whom it was collected.

Each handoff or transfer of the specimen must be documented, typically including the person's name receiving the specimen, the date and time, and the purpose of the transfer. This documented trail allows for the tracking of the specimen at any stage and confirms its secure handling and that there's been no tampering or misidentification.

Think of chain of custody as a well-detailed diary for each specimen. The diary details who collected it, who transported it, who received it, who analyzed it, what was done to it, and where it was stored or disposed of. This diary's entries protect the validity of the testing and the integrity of the specimen, ensuring that the test results are indisputably linked to the correct individual.

The chain of custody is a practice of precision and responsibility, a cornerstone in building trust in laboratory processes and their results. Therefore, understanding and maintaining a strict chain of custody protocol is not just a nice-to-have but an absolute must-have for any phlebotomist.

Accidents happen, right? A sudden slip, a knock, or an unexpected imbalance, and the next thing you know, you're dealing with a spill or breakage of specimens during transportation. It's a scenario we all want to avoid, but if it does happen, it's crucial to handle it with caution and composure.

1. **Protection is key:** The first thing you should do is protect yourself and others around you. Put on appropriate personal protective equipment (PPE) if you're not already wearing it - gloves, a lab coat, and face and eye protection.
2. **Isolate the area:** Barricade the area where the spill has occurred. This will keep unsuspecting individuals from wandering into the contaminated zone and reduce the chance of spreading the spill.
3. **Notify the necessary parties:** Inform your supervisor and other relevant personnel about the incident as soon as possible. The laboratory's spill management protocol will likely need to be initiated.
4. **Clean the spill:** Use a spill kit, if one is available. Start by placing absorbent material around the spill to prevent it from spreading further. Then, apply an appropriate disinfectant. Absorb the liquid again with fresh absorbent materials, and collect the materials in a biohazard bag. The disinfection process may need to be repeated depending on the nature of the spill.

5. **Dispose of the waste:** All waste materials, including broken glass, should be placed in a puncture-resistant biohazard container. Never try to pick up broken glass with your hands, even when wearing gloves - use a brush and dustpan.
6. **Follow up:** Document the incident per your facility's protocol and replace any damaged or depleted supplies.

Remember, safety comes first, and haste often leads to more accidents. A calm, collected, and careful approach will ensure that the spill is effectively and safely managed, protecting everyone in the facility.

Specimen processing, in the realm of a clinical laboratory, is a crucial bridge between specimen collection and actual testing. This integral phase involves preparing collected samples for analysis in a way that will render accurate and reliable test results.

The processing of a specimen depends on the type of test to be conducted and may involve several steps. These could include centrifugation, which separates different components of a specimen (like blood into plasma, buffy coat, and red blood cells); aliquoting, which is the process of dividing a specimen into smaller portions for multiple tests; or specific treatments to prepare the specimen, such as heating, chilling, or adding particular chemicals.

So, how does specimen processing differ from collection or testing? Well, specimen collection is the first step, where a sample is collected from a patient. This could be blood, urine, sputum, tissue, or any other biological sample. Strict protocols for collection must be followed to ensure the integrity and representativeness of the sample.

On the other hand, testing is the phase that comes after processing. Once a specimen has been appropriately processed, it's then analyzed for specific parameters, compounds, cells, or microorganisms according to the prescribed test methods.

The power of specimen processing, though, should not be underestimated! It is a vital link that directly influences the quality of the test results. Improper handling during processing can introduce errors, making it a critical part of the laboratory workflow that requires a high level of skill and meticulous attention to detail.

The processing of specimens in a clinical laboratory is a highly specialized and meticulous task. The goal is to prepare the collected samples appropriately for the various tests they will undergo. Let's look at the common steps involved in specimen processing and how these steps can vary based on the specimen type - blood, urine, or tissue.

For all specimens, the first step is to verify that the specimen is correctly labeled with patient identification and the date and time of collection. This ensures that the test results can be correctly attributed to the right patient. Next, any special handling requirements, such as protection from light or immediate chilling, should be attended to promptly.

1. **Blood Specimens:** After collection, blood specimens usually need to be centrifuged to separate the blood into different components. For example, a serum separator tube (SST) is first allowed to clot at room temperature and then centrifuged to separate the serum from the blood cells. Plasma specimens, collected in tubes with anticoagulants, are typically centrifuged immediately after gentle mixing. Once the blood components are separated, they can be aliquoted for different tests.
2. **Urine Specimens:** A fresh urine sample can be analyzed directly for some tests, such as urinalysis. For others, like culture and sensitivity, the specimen may need to be centrifuged and the sediment used. If testing isn't immediate, refrigeration is required to slow down the growth of any bacteria present.
3. **Tissue Specimens:** These samples require a different approach. Tissue specimens are usually fixed in a substance like formalin to preserve the tissue structure. Then, they undergo a series of processing steps that prepare them for embedding in paraffin wax blocks. Once the tissues are embedded, thin sections are cut using a microtome for examination under a microscope.

While the steps may vary somewhat based on the type of sample and the tests to be performed, the objective remains the same: to preserve the integrity of the specimen and ensure that it is in an optimal condition for accurate and reliable testing. Specimen processing is a critical step in the laboratory workflow, demanding precise technique and a solid understanding of how different handling practices can impact test results.

Centrifugation, a common step in the processing of many types of specimens, is crucial in preparing samples for analysis in the clinical laboratory. It utilizes the principle of sedimentation, where the centrifugal force causes heavier components in a mixture to move outward towards the periphery of the centrifuge tube, while lighter components move towards the center.

In the context of blood samples, centrifugation is employed to separate blood into its various components: plasma or serum, buffy coat (containing white blood cells and platelets), and red blood cells. This separation is vital for many tests that require specific components of the blood, such as chemistry assays performed on serum or plasma, or complete blood counts performed on whole blood.

Centrifugation is also commonly used in urine specimen processing, often to sediment solids for microscopic examination, or for microbiological cultures where it aids in concentrating organisms present.

However, performing centrifugation necessitates certain precautions:

1. **Balancing the Centrifuge:** Tubes of equal weight and volume need to be placed opposite each other in the centrifuge. This is crucial for maintaining balance when the centrifuge is in operation. Imbalance can damage the centrifuge and potentially pose a safety risk.
2. **Tube Securement:** Tubes should be properly secured in the centrifuge to prevent them from breaking or opening during the process, which could lead to potential aerosol hazards.

3. **Setting the Right Speed and Time:** The centrifugation speed (revolutions per minute or RPM) and time need to be set according to the requirements of the specific test. Over or under centrifugation can adversely affect the quality of the sample and the test results.
4. **Handling Post Centrifugation:** Once centrifugation is complete, the tubes should be carefully handled to avoid mixing the separated components. For example, when removing serum or plasma, a pipette should be used to gently aspirate the supernatant without disturbing the underlying cellular layer.

Remember, successful centrifugation aids in achieving accurate test results, but it demands meticulous attention to protocol and safe practices.

Aliquoting is a process in which a larger specimen is divided into smaller portions or 'aliquots'. This is a crucial step in specimen processing in a clinical laboratory setting for several reasons. First, it allows multiple tests to be run on the same sample while keeping the original specimen intact. Second, it provides a means for distributing the sample to various sections of the laboratory. Third, aliquoting is key for sample storage and future testing, if required.

The following steps describe a typical procedure for aliquoting a sample:
1. **Identify the Sample**: Always ensure you are working with the correct sample by double-checking the sample ID. Misidentification of samples can lead to serious errors.
2. **Prepare Aliquots**: Using a clean, single-use pipette or mechanical pipettor, gently aspirate the required amount of sample. It's crucial to avoid touching the inside of the sample container to prevent contamination.
3. **Transfer to Aliquot Tubes**: Carefully dispense the aspirated sample into the correctly labeled aliquot tube. If the specimen is a biological fluid (like serum or plasma), avoid disturbing any sediment or the cellular layer.
4. **Label Aliquots**: Each aliquot tube must be accurately and clearly labeled with the sample ID, the date/time of aliquoting, and the initials of the person performing the aliquoting. The labels should adhere well to the tubes and remain legible in the conditions where the samples will be stored.
5. **Cap and Store Aliquots**: Securely cap the aliquot tubes and store them as per the sample's required storage conditions.
6. **Documentation**: Accurately record the process, noting the sample ID, the volume of each aliquot, the number of aliquots made, and the storage location.

Aliquoting requires meticulous attention to prevent contamination, ensure accuracy, and maintain sample integrity. With careful and precise work, it's an invaluable tool in the effective processing of specimens in the clinical laboratory.

Correct data entry during specimen processing is absolutely critical to ensure accurate test results and proper patient care. The information entered into the laboratory information system (LIS) serves as the primary way to track and identify specimens, link results to the right patient, and enable effective communication between laboratory professionals and healthcare providers. Mistakes in data entry can lead to misidentification of samples, incorrect test results being reported, or potentially harmful treatment decisions.

During specimen processing, the following key pieces of information are typically entered into the LIS:

1. **Patient Identification Information**: This includes the patient's full name, date of birth, gender, and a unique identifier like a patient ID number or medical record number.
2. **Specimen Information**: This refers to the type of specimen collected (e.g., blood, urine), the date and time of collection, and any special conditions related to the sample (e.g., fasting, postprandial).
3. **Requested Tests**: The specific tests or panels of tests ordered by the healthcare provider should be carefully entered.
4. **Phlebotomist Identification**: The person who collected the specimen should be identified in case of any issues or questions regarding the collection procedure.
5. **Specimen Condition**: If there were any issues with the specimen (e.g., hemolysis in a blood sample, insufficient volume), these should be noted.
6. **Processing Information**: This includes the time of receipt in the lab, the time of processing, and any steps taken during processing like centrifugation or aliquoting.
7. **Distribution Information**: The location or department where the specimen was sent for testing should be recorded.

It's important to remember that data entry isn't a one-time task - it's an ongoing process that continues through the testing and reporting stages. Regularly reviewing and updating the information in the LIS as needed helps to maintain a strong link between the patient, the specimen, and the test results, ensuring that healthcare providers have accurate and timely information for making diagnostic and treatment decisions.

During specimen processing, several potential errors can arise which could significantly impact test results and subsequent patient care. Let's explore these errors and how phlebotomists can contribute to preventing them.

1. **Misidentification**: One of the most critical errors is specimen misidentification. If samples are not correctly identified with the patient's information, it can lead to severe consequences, including wrong diagnosis and treatment.

Prevention: Phlebotomists can contribute to preventing this error by correctly labeling specimens immediately after collection, in the presence of the patient, to ensure the right patient is linked to the right sample.

2. **Inadequate Specimen Quality**: Errors can also occur when the specimen is of poor quality due to hemolysis, contamination, or improper handling during collection.

Prevention: By using correct collection techniques, phlebotomists can ensure the quality of the specimen. Proper handling and storage post-collection are also essential to maintain specimen integrity.

3. **Processing Delays**: The time between specimen collection and processing can impact the quality of some specimens, potentially affecting test results.

Prevention: Phlebotomists can play a role by transporting samples to the lab as quickly as possible and providing clear instructions about any time-sensitive handling requirements.

4. **Data Entry Errors**: Mistakes in data entry during specimen processing can lead to a miscommunication of results.

Prevention: Although phlebotomists may not be directly involved in data entry during processing, they can ensure correct and legible information on specimen labels and requisition forms to prevent misunderstandings or mistakes during entry.

5. **Improper Storage**: The inappropriate storage of specimens can degrade the samples, leading to inaccurate test results.

Prevention: Phlebotomists should be aware of and adhere to storage requirements for different types of samples, such as necessary refrigeration or protection from light.

6. **Cross-Contamination**: If specimens are not handled correctly, there's a risk of cross-contamination.

Prevention: Phlebotomists can prevent this by using new, sterile equipment for each collection, properly disposing of used supplies, and adhering to infection control practices.

Through their direct involvement in specimen collection and their understanding of the entire testing process, phlebotomists are well-positioned to help prevent these errors and contribute to the overall quality of patient care.

Quality control (QC) in the specimen processing area is vital to ensure the reliability and accuracy of test results. It encompasses a set of procedures designed to monitor the quality of all aspects related to the processing of samples. Here are some key quality control measures:

1. **Standard Operating Procedures (SOPs)**: One of the primary QC measures is to have detailed, written SOPs that clearly define every step of the specimen processing procedure, including collection, handling, storage, and transportation. These should be followed precisely to reduce errors and maintain the integrity of the sample.

2. **Quality Control Samples**: These are samples with known values that are used to ensure that the testing system is working correctly. By comparing the test results from these control samples with their known values, laboratories can verify that their processes are accurate and reliable.

3. **Proficiency Testing**: This is a type of external QC where samples from an outside agency are processed and tested by the lab to ensure that they're performing analyses correctly and their results are comparable to other laboratories.

4. **Equipment Calibration and Maintenance**: Regular calibration and maintenance of equipment such as centrifuges, refrigerators, and freezers are crucial. This ensures that they are functioning correctly, maintaining the appropriate conditions necessary for specimen integrity.

5. **Training and Competency Assessment**: Regular training and assessment of staff competency ensure that everyone involved in specimen processing is up to date with the procedures and capable of performing their tasks accurately.

6. **Error Tracking and Continuous Improvement**: Any errors or incidents should be recorded and reviewed to identify trends, areas for improvement, and implement corrective actions. This continuous improvement approach contributes to reducing errors and enhancing the overall quality of specimen processing.

7. **Environmental Conditions**: Regular monitoring of environmental conditions, such as temperature and humidity in the processing and storage areas, helps maintain the integrity of the samples.

These quality control measures together ensure that the entire process from sample collection to testing is controlled and reliable. This, in turn, ensures that the test results are accurate and reliable, leading to correct diagnoses and effective treatment plans for patients.

Proper maintenance and cleaning of equipment used in specimen processing is critical to maintaining laboratory safety and quality assurance. Here are the key procedures to keep in mind:

1. **Regular Maintenance and Calibration**: All laboratory equipment, including centrifuges, pipettes, refrigerators, freezers, and analyzers, should be serviced and calibrated on a regular schedule as per the manufacturer's instructions. This not only ensures accurate and reliable test results but also extends the life of the equipment.

2. **Daily Inspections**: Routine inspections can help catch issues early before they affect test results. Each day, staff should check equipment for any visible signs of wear and tear or malfunctions.

3. **Proper Cleaning**: Each piece of equipment will have specific cleaning procedures outlined by the manufacturer. Typically, this includes cleaning after each use to prevent cross-contamination between samples, as well as a more thorough cleaning at regular intervals.

4. **Correct Use of Equipment**: Using equipment in a manner consistent with its design and purpose also helps to maintain it. Misuse can lead to damage and inaccurate results.

5. **Documentation**: Keep detailed records of all maintenance, cleaning, and calibration activities. This helps to track the equipment's performance over time and is necessary for auditing purposes.

6. **Safety Practices**: Always use appropriate personal protective equipment (PPE) when handling and cleaning laboratory equipment. Follow all safety guidelines to protect staff from potential hazards associated with the use and cleaning of the equipment.

By implementing these procedures, a laboratory ensures its equipment is in optimal working condition, which leads to accurate and reliable results. It also minimizes potential hazards, creating a safer working environment. Therefore, these procedures directly contribute to both laboratory safety and quality assurance.

Exam Prep Section:

Welcome to the Practice Exam section of your study guide! This portion of the guide is designed to provide you with an opportunity to test your knowledge, reinforce the concepts you have learned, and help you identify any areas that may require additional study.

Each question in this section is followed immediately by its answer and a detailed explanation. Why is it structured this way, you may ask?

The rationale behind placing the answer and explanation immediately after the question is based on principles of effective learning and retention. When you read a question, your brain starts to process the information and formulates an answer. Providing the correct answer and explanation immediately after allows you to confirm your understanding right away, correct any misconceptions, and reinforce the learning process.

Immediate feedback is a powerful learning tool. It allows for immediate correction if you answered incorrectly, helping to avoid the reinforcement of incorrect information. It also provides an opportunity for you to understand the reasoning behind the correct answer, improving your grasp of the underlying concepts.

We also understand that while taking a practice exam, the flow of thought should not be interrupted by having to navigate to the back of the book to check answers. We want to make your study process as smooth and productive as possible.

As you work through these practice questions, remember that it's not just about getting the right answer. It's also about understanding why an answer is correct, and why others are not. This deep understanding is what will truly prepare you for success.

So, take a deep breath, stay focused, and let's begin the journey towards acing your examination!

1. In a clinical lab setting, what is the most effective way to protect oneself from infectious diseases?
a) Use of gloves and face masks only when handling specimens.
b) Regular handwashing and avoiding touching the face.
c) Keeping the laboratory doors and windows open for ventilation.
d) Eating a balanced diet to boost the immune system.

Answer: b. Hand hygiene is one of the most effective ways to prevent the spread of infections. While gloves provide a physical barrier, they can still be contaminated and spread pathogens if not used properly. Therefore, handwashing, especially after removing gloves, and avoiding touching the face are critical. The other options, while may be important in certain contexts, are not the most effective ways to prevent infection in a laboratory setting.

2. A laboratory worker spills a chemical on their skin. What should be their immediate action?
a) Rinse the affected area with running water.
b) Wipe the area with a dry cloth.
c) Apply an antidote to neutralize the chemical.
d) Continue working, as long as there is no pain.

Answer: a. Immediate rinsing with running water is recommended to flush the chemical out and minimize skin damage. Other actions may be required depending on the chemical, but rinsing with water should be the first step. The other options may not effectively mitigate harm and could even exacerbate the situation.

3. Which of the following best describes the principle of Universal Precautions in the clinical laboratory?
a) All specimens should be considered potentially hazardous.
b) Only specimens from patients with known infections should be considered hazardous.
c) Universal precautions are not necessary if the worker has been vaccinated.
d) Universal precautions should only be applied to blood and body fluid specimens.

Answer: A. Universal precautions dictate that all patient specimens should be treated as if they are infectious, regardless of the patient's known or suspected disease status. This is to protect healthcare workers from pathogens that may be present, even if the patient has not been diagnosed with a communicable disease.

4. If an incident like a needlestick injury occurs in the laboratory, what is the first thing an employee should do?
a) Continue working and report the incident at the end of the shift.
b) Clean the wound, report to the supervisor, and fill out an incident report.
c) Wait for symptoms to develop before taking any action.
d) Take a break to recover from the shock.

Answer: b. Following a needlestick injury, the wound should be cleaned immediately. Prompt reporting to a supervisor is crucial so that risk assessment can be done and appropriate post-exposure prophylaxis can be initiated if needed. An incident report must also be filled out for record-keeping and for assessment of workplace safety.

5. Why is it important to wear personal protective equipment (PPE) correctly in a laboratory setting?
a) To look professional and organized.
b) To protect against potential exposure to hazardous materials and infectious agents.
c) Because it is a legal requirement and failure to do so can lead to penalties.
d) To intimidate the patients and establish authority.

Answer: b. The primary purpose of PPE is to protect the wearer from exposure to hazards, including chemicals, infectious agents, and physical injuries. While legal compliance is important, the primary reason to wear PPE is for personal safety.

6. Why is it necessary to segregate biomedical waste in the clinical laboratory?
a) To increase the volume of waste.
b) To ensure the safety of personnel and environment.
c) To make the laboratory look more organized.
d) It is not really necessary; it's just a good practice.

Answer: b Segregating biomedical waste is essential for the safety of personnel and the environment. It ensures that hazardous waste is properly handled, treated, and disposed of, reducing the risk of injury and contamination.

7. A specimen container is marked with a biohazard symbol. What does this symbol indicate?
a) The container holds a non-hazardous substance.
b) The container must be handled with universal precautions.
c) The container should be recycled.
d) The container should be refrigerated.

Answer: b A biohazard symbol indicates that the contents of the container may pose an infection risk, and hence, should be handled with universal precautions to prevent exposure to potentially infectious materials.

8. What type of fire extinguisher should be used on an electrical fire in the lab?
a) Water fire extinguisher.
b) Carbon dioxide or dry chemical fire extinguisher.
c) Foam fire extinguisher.
d) Any type of fire extinguisher will work.

Answer: b For electrical fires (classified as Class C fires in the US or Class E in Australia), a non-conductive extinguishing agent such as carbon dioxide (CO_2) or a dry chemical should be used. Using water or foam could potentially cause electrocution.

9. How frequently should safety equipment (such as fire extinguishers, fume hoods, and eye wash stations) in the laboratory be inspected?
a) Annually.
b) Monthly.
c) Whenever a problem is suspected.
d) Every five years.

Answer: b. Regular checks, typically on a monthly basis, are crucial to ensure that safety equipment is in good working condition and ready to use in the event of an emergency. While inspections may also occur annually, frequent checks are important to catch any problems early.

10. What is the primary purpose of the Material Safety Data Sheet (MSDS) in the laboratory?
a) To provide procedures for laboratory tests.
b) To provide information about the chemical, its hazards, and measures for its safe handling.
c) To provide a list of all laboratory employees.
d) To provide a guide for the maintenance of laboratory equipment.

Answer: b MSDS, also known as Safety Data Sheet (SDS), provides comprehensive information about a specific chemical - including its physical and chemical properties, potential health hazards, safe handling and storage procedures, emergency procedures, and disposal considerations. This ensures safety in the workplace and is a vital resource in case of a spill or exposure.

11. You are a laboratory technician working in a clinical lab. Which of the following is the best practice when dealing with potentially infectious specimens?
a) Handling all specimens with bare hands to feel the consistency
b) Considering all specimens as potentially infectious
c) Using the same gloves for all specimens to reduce waste
d) Not wearing a lab coat to stay comfortable

Answer: b) Considering all specimens as potentially infectious. Explanation: Universal precautions suggest that all specimens should be treated as if they could potentially be infectious, regardless of the patient's known disease state. This ensures maximum safety and reduces the risk of contamination or infection.

12. A lab worker splashes a potentially infectious liquid onto their skin. What should they do immediately?
a) Continue working and wash the area later
b) Rinse the area with water and then apply an antiseptic
c) Ignore it because the skin acts as a natural barrier to infection
d) Immediately leave the lab without taking any action

Answer: b) Rinse the area with water and then apply an antiseptic. Explanation: If a lab worker gets a potentially infectious substance on their skin, it should be washed off immediately with water and an antiseptic, if available. Immediate action is crucial to prevent the risk of infection.

13. In the event of a small chemical spill in the lab, who is primarily responsible for initiating the cleanup?
a) The lab manager
b) The person who caused the spill
c) Any available lab technician
d) An external cleaning service

Answer: b) The person who caused the spill. Explanation: The person who caused the spill is typically responsible for initiating the cleanup, provided they can do so safely. They should be trained in how to handle such incidents, including using appropriate personal protective equipment (PPE) and spill kits.

14. When should a healthcare worker perform hand hygiene?
a) Only before eating meals
b) After every patient interaction, regardless of contact
c) Only when their hands look dirty
d) At the end of their shift

Answer: b) After every patient interaction, regardless of contact. Explanation: Hand hygiene is an essential measure to prevent healthcare-associated infections and the spread of antimicrobial resistance. It should be performed after every patient interaction, regardless of whether physical contact was made or not.

15. Which of the following statements about the use of personal protective equipment (PPE) is correct?
a) PPE should be shared between colleagues to conserve resources
b) PPE should be used only in emergencies
c) PPE should be chosen based on the anticipated exposure
d) PPE is uncomfortable, so its use should be minimized

Answer: c) PPE should be chosen based on the anticipated exposure. Explanation: PPE should be selected specifically based on the degree of anticipated exposure to infectious material. Different tasks and procedures may require different types of PPE, and it is essential to choose the correct type for each situation to ensure maximum protection.

16. What is the primary reason for decontaminating work surfaces in the lab?
a) To make the lab look cleaner
b) To prevent potential infections
c) To kill all living organisms on the surface
d) To make surfaces shiny

Answer: b) To prevent potential infections. Explanation: Decontamination of work surfaces is done primarily to prevent the spread of infections. While it may have aesthetic benefits like making the lab look cleaner, the main goal is to reduce the risk of spreading potential pathogens.

17. Which of the following actions is appropriate if you are unable to interpret a safety data sheet (SDS)?
a) Ignore the SDS and continue your work
b) Ask a colleague for their interpretation
c) Consult with a supervisor or safety officer
d) Guess the meaning of the SDS and proceed with your work

Answer: c) Consult with a supervisor or safety officer. Explanation: If you're unsure about interpreting any part of a Safety Data Sheet (SDS), you should consult with your supervisor or a safety officer. Incorrect interpretation can lead to unsafe handling of substances, so it's important to get accurate information.

18. Which of the following practices is essential in preventing laboratory-acquired infections?
a) Frequent breaks to rest
b) Personal calls during work hours
c) Adherence to standard precautions
d) Unrestricted food and drink in the lab

Answer: c) Adherence to standard precautions. Explanation: Standard precautions are a set of infection control practices that healthcare workers use to treat all patients, regardless of their presumed infection status. They include hand hygiene, use of PPE, safe injection practices, safe handling of potentially contaminated equipment, and respiratory hygiene.

19. What is the best practice for disposing of sharp objects like needles and scalpel blades in a healthcare setting?
a) Throw them in the regular trash can
b) Place them in a rigid, puncture-resistant sharps container
c) Wrap them in a paper towel before disposing of them in the regular trash can
d) Wash them thoroughly and then place them in a regular trash can

Answer: b) Place them in a rigid, puncture-resistant sharps container. Explanation: Used sharp objects like needles and blades should always be disposed of in a designated sharps container. These containers are specifically designed to be puncture-resistant and leak-proof to prevent injuries and exposure to potential infections.

20. What should a lab worker do if they notice a safety hazard in their workspace?
a) Ignore it and hope it goes away
b) Try to fix it themselves without any guidance
c) Report it to their supervisor immediately
d) Wait for the monthly safety inspection for it to be found

Answer: c) Report it to their supervisor immediately. Explanation: Safety hazards should never be ignored or left to be discovered later. They should be reported immediately to a supervisor or safety officer to ensure they are handled properly and promptly, minimizing the risk of accidents or injuries.

21. Standard precautions in a healthcare setting refer to:
a) Guidelines to be used only when dealing with patients with confirmed infections
b) Practices that should be applied universally, regardless of suspected or confirmed infection
c) Steps that only senior staff members need to follow
d) A set of optional suggestions to follow if time permits

Answer: b) Practices that should be applied universally, regardless of suspected or confirmed infection. Explanation: Standard precautions are a group of infection control practices that healthcare workers use for the care of all patients, regardless of their presumed infection status. It includes hand hygiene, use of personal protective equipment, and safe handling of potentially contaminated equipment or surfaces.

22. When should hand hygiene be performed in the healthcare setting?
a) Only after direct patient contact
b) Before and after every patient interaction, after contact with body fluids, and after contact with patient surroundings
c) Only at the beginning and end of a healthcare worker's shift
d) Once a day to save on resources

Answer: b) Before and after every patient interaction, after contact with body fluids, and after contact with patient surroundings. Explanation: Hand hygiene is a crucial element of standard precautions and should be performed before and after every patient interaction, after contact with body fluids, and after contact with any surface in the patient's surroundings.

23. What type of personal protective equipment (PPE) should be used when performing a procedure that is likely to generate splashes of blood or body fluids?
a) Gloves only
b) Mask and gloves only
c) Goggles, gloves, gown, and mask
d) No PPE is required as long as you're careful

Answer: c) Goggles, gloves, gown, and mask. Explanation: Standard precautions dictate that for procedures that may generate splashes of blood or body fluids, full barrier protection (which includes gloves, gowns, masks, and goggles or face shields) should be used to protect against potential exposure.

24. What is the recommended method for disposing of sharp items like needles in a healthcare setting?
a) Disposing of them in a regular waste bin
b) Placing them directly in a puncture-resistant sharps container
c) Washing them and then reusing them
d) Placing them in a plastic bag before disposing of them in a regular waste bin

Answer: b) Placing them directly in a puncture-resistant sharps container. Explanation: Used sharp objects like needles should be immediately disposed of in a designated, puncture-resistant sharps container. This prevents needlestick injuries and potential exposure to infections.

25. What should be done if a healthcare worker gets blood or other potentially infectious materials in their eyes?
a) They should wait until their break to wash their eyes
b) They should immediately irrigate their eyes with water or saline
c) They should rub their eyes to try to remove the material
d) They should continue working and wash their eyes later

Answer: b) They should immediately irrigate their eyes with water or saline. Explanation: If blood or other potentially infectious materials get into the eyes, it's important to act quickly. The eyes should be immediately irrigated with clean water or saline to remove the material and reduce the chance of infection.

26. Which of the following is not a part of standard precautions in healthcare?
a) Use of personal protective equipment
b) Hand hygiene
c) Recycling used needles
d) Safe injection practices

Answer: c) Recycling used needles. Explanation: Recycling used needles is not a part of standard precautions and is actually a violation of these precautions. Used needles should be immediately disposed of in a designated, puncture-resistant sharps container.

27. Respiratory hygiene/cough etiquette is a part of standard precautions and includes:
a) Coughing into the open air to spread germs away from the body
b) Covering the mouth and nose with a tissue when coughing or sneezing, and proper disposal of the tissue
c) Reusing tissues for multiple sneezes to conserve resources
d) Suppressing all coughs and sneezes to prevent the spread of germs

Answer: b) Covering the mouth and nose with a tissue when coughing or sneezing, and proper disposal of the tissue. Explanation: Respiratory hygiene/cough etiquette is an integral part of standard precautions and includes covering the mouth and nose with a tissue (or the elbow if a tissue isn't available) when coughing or sneezing, followed by hand hygiene and proper disposal of tissues.

28. Who do standard precautions apply to in the healthcare setting?
a) Only to healthcare workers
b) Only to patients
c) To healthcare workers, patients, and visitors
d) Only to individuals with a known infection

Answer: c) To healthcare workers, patients, and visitors. Explanation: Standard precautions apply to all individuals in a healthcare setting, including healthcare workers, patients, and visitors, regardless of their suspected or confirmed infection status.

29. What is the primary goal of standard precautions?
a) To prevent healthcare workers from getting sick
b) To reduce the risk of transmission of microorganisms from both recognized and unrecognized sources of infection in healthcare settings
c) To reduce the amount of cleaning that needs to be done in healthcare settings
d) To make healthcare settings appear safer to visitors

Answer: b) To reduce the risk of transmission of microorganisms from both recognized and unrecognized sources of infection in healthcare settings. Explanation: The primary goal of standard precautions is to reduce the risk of transmission of microorganisms from both recognized and unrecognized sources of infection in healthcare settings. This is done through a combination of hand hygiene, use of personal protective equipment, respiratory hygiene, and safe injection practices, among other measures.

30. What is the main purpose of wearing Personal Protective Equipment (PPE) in a healthcare setting?
a) To make the healthcare provider more comfortable
b) To protect the healthcare provider and the patient from infectious diseases
c) To provide a barrier against harmful chemicals
d) To make the healthcare provider more visible to patients

Answer: b) To protect the healthcare provider and the patient from infectious diseases. Explanation: Personal Protective Equipment (PPE) is worn in healthcare settings to provide a barrier between healthcare workers and potential infectious materials, thereby protecting both the healthcare workers and the patients they care for.

31. When is it necessary to wear a mask in a healthcare setting?
a) Only when dealing with patients with known respiratory diseases
b) During all patient care
c) Only during surgical procedures
d) When working in a setting where airborne precautions are necessary, or when certain procedures are performed that may generate splashes or sprays of body fluids

Answer: d) When working in a setting where airborne precautions are necessary, or when certain procedures are performed that may generate splashes or sprays of body fluids. Explanation: A mask should be worn in healthcare settings where airborne precautions are in place (for diseases that are spread through the air), and during procedures that may generate splashes or sprays of body fluids to protect the healthcare worker's nose and mouth from potential exposure.

32. Which of the following is a necessary step when donning (putting on) PPE?
a) Putting on gloves before gown
b) Wearing personal eyeglasses instead of goggles for eye protection
c) Performing hand hygiene before donning the PPE
d) Touching the outside of the gown while removing it

Answer: c) Performing hand hygiene before donning the PPE. Explanation: Performing hand hygiene is a critical step before putting on PPE. This prevents the transfer of microorganisms from the hands to the PPE, and subsequently, to the patient.

33. Why is the order in which PPE is removed important?
a) It is not important; PPE can be removed in any order
b) It minimizes the risk of self-contamination
c) It maximizes the efficiency of healthcare workers
d) It ensures the PPE can be reused

Answer: b) It minimizes the risk of self-contamination. Explanation: The order in which PPE is removed is designed to minimize the risk of self-contamination by ensuring the areas of PPE that are most contaminated are removed first and in a way that prevents the spread of infectious material.

34. What should healthcare workers do if their gloves get torn during a procedure?
a) Continue the procedure and change the gloves afterwards
b) Remove the gloves, perform hand hygiene, and put on a new pair of gloves
c) Use medical tape to fix the tear
d) Remove only the torn glove and replace it with a new one

Answer: b) Remove the gloves, perform hand hygiene, and put on a new pair of gloves. Explanation: If gloves are torn during a procedure, they no longer provide effective protection. The healthcare worker should remove the gloves, perform hand hygiene, and put on a new pair of gloves to continue the procedure.

35. Which PPE item is considered the final barrier against the transmission of infection?
a) Gown
b) Gloves
c) Mask
d) Face shield

Answer: b) Gloves. Explanation: Gloves are the final barrier against transmission. They are often the last piece of PPE to be donned and the first to be removed. Therefore, proper handling of gloves is critical to minimize contamination risk.

36. What should a healthcare worker do with their PPE after finishing a procedure with a patient who has a suspected or confirmed infection?
a) Leave the PPE in the patient's room for cleaning staff to collect
b) Remove and dispose of the PPE in the appropriate trash bin
c) Reuse the PPE for the next patient to conserve supplies
d) Take the PPE home for washing

Answer: b) Remove and dispose of the PPE in the appropriate trash bin. Explanation: PPE should be promptly removed after finishing a procedure and disposed of in the appropriate trash bin in the healthcare facility. Reusing or improperly disposing of PPE can lead to the spread of infection.

37. How often should PPE be changed?
a) Only when it becomes visibly dirty
b) After every patient encounter
c) Every 5 hours, regardless of patient contact
d) Once a week

Answer: b) After every patient encounter. Explanation: PPE should be changed after every patient encounter to prevent cross-contamination between patients. This includes gloves, gowns, masks, and eye protection.

38. What PPE should be used when there is a risk of splashes or sprays of body fluids?
a) Gloves only
b) Gloves and gown
c) Gloves, gown, and mask
d) Gloves, gown, mask, and eye protection

Answer: d) Gloves, gown, mask, and eye protection. Explanation: When there is a risk of splashes or sprays of body fluids, comprehensive PPE should be used to protect the healthcare worker. This includes gloves to protect the hands, a gown to protect clothing and exposed skin, a mask to protect the nose and mouth, and eye protection to shield the eyes.

39. Which of the following should you do if you accidentally stick yourself with a used needle?
a) Continue working; it's not a big deal
b) Immediately wash the area with soap and water, then report the incident to your supervisor
c) Put a bandage on the wound and don't tell anyone
d) Try to draw blood to clean out the wound

Answer: b) Immediately wash the area with soap and water, then report the incident to your supervisor. Explanation: After a needlestick or sharps injury, you should immediately wash the area with soap and water and then report the incident to your supervisor. It's essential to follow these steps to prevent potential infection and to ensure appropriate follow-up measures are taken.

40. Where should used needles be disposed of in a healthcare setting?
a) In the regular trash
b) In a designated sharps container
c) In a plastic bag
d) In the recycling bin

Answer: b) In a designated sharps container. Explanation: Used needles and other sharps should always be disposed of in a designated sharps container. These containers are specifically designed to safely contain and store sharps to prevent injuries and reduce the risk of infection.

41. What should be done with a sharps container when it becomes three-quarters full?
a) Continue using it until it is completely full
b) Seal it and dispose of it in the regular trash
c) Seal it and dispose of it according to facility guidelines for sharps waste
d) Empty it and reuse it

Answer: c) Seal it and dispose of it according to facility guidelines for sharps waste. Explanation: When a sharps container is about three-quarters full, it should be sealed and disposed of according to the facility's guidelines for sharps waste. This practice prevents overfilling, which could lead to sharps injuries.

42. Which of the following is a safe practice for handling sharps?
a) Recapping needles after use
b) Passing sharps directly to another person
c) Disposing of sharps in a designated sharps container
d) Leaving sharps on a patient's bedside table

Answer: c) Disposing of sharps in a designated sharps container. Explanation: Sharps should always be disposed of in a designated sharps container immediately after use. Recapping needles, passing sharps directly to another person, or leaving sharps unattended are all unsafe practices that increase the risk of sharps injuries.

43. What is the primary reason for using safety-engineered sharp devices in healthcare settings?
a) They are less expensive
b) They reduce the risk of sharps injuries
c) They are more efficient
d) They can be reused

Answer: b) They reduce the risk of sharps injuries. Explanation: Safety-engineered sharp devices have built-in safety features that help to reduce the risk of sharps injuries. These can include retractable needles, sheaths that cover the sharp after use, or mechanisms that prevent re-use.

44. Why is it important not to recap needles after use?
a) It's a waste of time
b) It's difficult to do
c) It increases the risk of a needlestick injury
d) It damages the needle

Answer: c) It increases the risk of a needlestick injury. Explanation: Recapping needles after use increases the risk of a needlestick injury, as the healthcare worker may accidentally stick themselves with the used needle. Instead, used needles should be immediately disposed of in a sharps container.

45. How should sharps be carried from one place to another in a healthcare setting?
a) In your hand, with the sharp end pointing down
b) In a designated sharps container
c) In a plastic bag
d) In your pocket

Answer: b) In a designated sharps container. Explanation: Sharps should never be carried in your hand, in a plastic bag, or in your pocket, as these practices increase the risk of sharps injuries. Instead, they should be placed in a designated sharps container and carried in the container.

46. What should you do if a sharps container is not readily available?
a) Leave the sharp on a flat surface until a container is available
b) Dispose of the sharp in the regular trash
c) Carry the sharp with you until you find a container
d) Store the sharp safely and temporarily, then transfer it to a sharps container as soon as possible

Answer: d) Store the sharp safely and temporarily, then transfer it to a sharps container as soon as possible. Explanation: If a sharps container is not readily available, the sharp should be stored safely and temporarily (for example, in a hard-sided, puncture-resistant container) until it can be transferred to a sharps container.

47. Which of the following should you do if you find a used needle on the floor?
a) Pick it up with your hands and dispose of it in the regular trash
b) Leave it and notify cleaning staff
c) Pick it up with a mechanical device or gloved hands and dispose of it in a sharps container
d) Kick it to the side so nobody steps on it

Answer: c) Pick it up with a mechanical device or gloved hands and dispose of it in a sharps container. Explanation: If you find a used needle on the floor, you should pick it up using a mechanical device (like tongs or a brush and dustpan) or with gloved hands, taking care to avoid the sharp end. Then, dispose of it immediately in a sharps container.

48. Which of the following correctly defines Standard Precautions in healthcare?
a) Guidelines designed to protect patients from healthcare workers
b) Procedures only applied when treating patients known to have infectious diseases
c) A set of infection control practices used to prevent transmission of diseases
d) Practices used only in surgery and other invasive procedures

Answer: c) A set of infection control practices used to prevent transmission of diseases. Explanation: Standard Precautions are infection control practices used in healthcare to prevent transmission of diseases that can be acquired by contact with blood, body fluids, non-intact skin (including rashes), and mucous membranes.

49. Why are Standard Precautions considered essential in phlebotomy?
a) They prevent needlestick injuries
b) They protect both healthcare workers and patients from infectious diseases
c) They make the phlebotomy procedure faster
d) They are required by law in all states

Answer: b) They protect both healthcare workers and patients from infectious diseases. Explanation: Standard Precautions are essential in phlebotomy because they help protect both the healthcare worker and the patient from potential exposure to infectious diseases.

50. What is the primary purpose of hand hygiene in the context of Standard Precautions?
a) It's a routine procedure to be followed by healthcare workers
b) It prevents transmission of pathogens
c) It's only necessary when hands are visibly dirty
d) It's to make patients feel comfortable

Answer: b) It prevents transmission of pathogens. Explanation: Hand hygiene is a vital part of Standard Precautions because it helps to prevent the transmission of pathogens, including those that can lead to healthcare-associated infections.

51. In the context of Standard Precautions, when should personal protective equipment (PPE) be worn?
a) Only when treating patients known to have infectious diseases
b) At all times while in the healthcare facility
c) Whenever exposure to blood, body fluids, or other potentially infectious materials is likely
d) Only during invasive procedures

Answer: c) Whenever exposure to blood, body fluids, or other potentially infectious materials is likely. Explanation: According to Standard Precautions, personal protective equipment (PPE) should be worn whenever there's a potential for exposure to blood, body fluids, secretions, excretions, mucous membranes, or non-intact skin.

52. How should potentially contaminated surfaces be cleaned in accordance with Standard Precautions?
a) With soap and water only
b) With an EPA-registered disinfectant or a bleach solution
c) With alcohol-based hand sanitizer
d) With hot water only

Answer: b) With an EPA-registered disinfectant or a bleach solution. Explanation: According to Standard Precautions, surfaces that are likely to be contaminated with pathogens (including those in blood and body fluids) should be cleaned and disinfected with an EPA-registered disinfectant or a bleach solution.

53. What are droplet precautions?
a) Measures taken to prevent the spread of diseases that can be spread through the air over long distances
b) Measures taken to prevent the spread of diseases that can be spread through direct skin-to-skin contact
c) Measures taken to prevent the spread of diseases that can be spread through droplets in the air
d) Measures taken to prevent the spread of diseases that can be spread through blood and body fluids

Answer: c) Measures taken to prevent the spread of diseases that can be spread through droplets in the air. Explanation: Droplet precautions are a type of Standard Precaution designed to reduce the risk of transmission of pathogens spread through close respiratory or mucous membrane contact with respiratory secretions.

54. What is the most effective way to prevent healthcare-associated infections according to Standard Precautions?
a) Use of personal protective equipment (PPE)
b) Hand hygiene
c) Vaccination of healthcare workers
d) Use of antibiotics

Answer: b) Hand hygiene. Explanation: Hand hygiene is considered the most effective method of preventing healthcare-associated infections, according to Standard Precautions.

55. According to Standard Precautions, what should be done immediately after a needlestick injury?
a) Wash the area with soap and water, then report the incident
b) Apply an antibiotic ointment and a bandage, then continue work
c) Ignore it unless it starts to look infected
d) Apply a bandage and report the incident at the end of the shift

Answer: a) Wash the area with soap and water, then report the incident. Explanation: Following a needlestick or other sharps injury, the area should be immediately washed with soap and water, and the incident should be promptly reported so that appropriate follow-up can occur.

56. What is one of the key principles of Standard Precautions?
a) Treat all blood and body fluids as potentially infectious
b) Use personal protective equipment (PPE) only when necessary
c) Perform hand hygiene only after direct patient contact
d) Disinfect all surfaces at the end of each shift

Answer: a) Treat all blood and body fluids as potentially infectious. Explanation: One of the key principles of Standard Precautions is that all blood, body fluids, secretions, excretions, non-intact skin, and mucous membranes may contain transmissible infectious agents and should be treated as such.

57. What should be the first step in donning Personal Protective Equipment (PPE) for a phlebotomy procedure?
a) Putting on a mask
b) Putting on gloves
c) Putting on a gown
d) Hand hygiene

Answer: d) Hand hygiene. Explanation: The first step in putting on PPE is performing hand hygiene. This step is vital to avoid contaminating the PPE when putting it on.

58. When donning PPE, what should be put on after performing hand hygiene and before putting on gloves?
a) Mask
b) Face shield
c) Gown
d) Shoe covers

Answer: c) Gown. Explanation: After performing hand hygiene, the next step in the donning procedure is to put on the gown, then the mask or respirator, and finally the gloves.

59. What is the proper order of donning PPE for a phlebotomy procedure?
a) Hand hygiene, gown, mask, gloves
b) Hand hygiene, mask, gown, gloves
c) Gown, hand hygiene, mask, gloves
d) Gown, mask, hand hygiene, gloves

Answer: a) Hand hygiene, gown, mask, gloves. Explanation: The correct sequence of donning PPE is first performing hand hygiene, then putting on the gown, followed by the mask or respirator, and finally the gloves.

60. Which PPE item should be removed first after finishing a phlebotomy procedure?
a) Gloves
b) Mask
c) Gown
d) Shoe covers

Answer: a) Gloves. Explanation: After a phlebotomy procedure, the gloves should be removed first as they are most likely to be contaminated. The gloves should be removed in a manner that avoids skin contact with the outer surface.

61. When removing PPE, what should be done after removing the gloves but before removing the gown?
a) Perform hand hygiene
b) Remove the mask
c) Put on a new pair of gloves
d) Leave the patient's room

Answer: a) Perform hand hygiene. Explanation: After removing the gloves, the next step is to perform hand hygiene before proceeding to remove the gown. This is to prevent any potential contamination that may have occurred during glove removal.

62. What should be the last step after removing all PPE?
a) Leave the patient's room
b) Dispose of the PPE in a designated container
c) Wash hands with soap and water
d) Put on a new pair of gloves

Answer: c) Wash hands with soap and water. Explanation: The last step after removing all PPE is to perform hand hygiene, ideally by washing hands with soap and water. This final step ensures any potential contamination during the removal process is cleaned off.

63. What is the proper technique for removing gloves?
a) Pulling them off from the wrist
b) Turning them inside out as they are removed
c) Pulling them off from the fingertips
d) Cutting them off with scissors

Answer: b) Turning them inside out as they are removed. Explanation: The correct technique for removing gloves involves turning them inside out as they are removed. This technique helps to contain any contamination on the gloves.

64. What is the correct order for removing PPE?
a) Gloves, hand hygiene, gown, mask, hand hygiene
b) Gloves, gown, hand hygiene, mask, hand hygiene
c) Mask, gown, gloves, hand hygiene
d) Gown, gloves, mask, hand hygiene

Answer: b) Gloves, gown, hand hygiene, mask, hand hygiene. Explanation: The correct sequence for removing PPE is to first remove the gloves, perform hand hygiene, then remove the gown, followed by the mask or respirator, and finally perform hand hygiene again.

65. Where should contaminated PPE be disposed of?
a) Regular trash bin
b) Designated infectious waste container
c) Recyclable container
d) Any container available

Answer: b) Designated infectious waste container. Explanation: Contaminated PPE should be disposed of in a designated infectious waste container to prevent the spread of infections.

66. What is the importance of performing hand hygiene after removing each piece of PPE?
a) It keeps the hands clean for the next patient
b) It removes any potential contamination acquired during the removal process
c) It moisturizes the hands
d) It is a requirement by the healthcare facility

Answer: b) It removes any potential contamination acquired during the removal process. Explanation: Performing hand hygiene after removing each piece of PPE helps to remove any potential contamination that may have been acquired during the removal process.

67. Which piece of Personal Protective Equipment (PPE) is critical when performing a phlebotomy procedure to protect the hands?
a) Goggles
b) Gloves
c) Gown
d) Mask

Answer: b) Gloves. Explanation: Gloves are a critical piece of PPE when performing a phlebotomy procedure as they protect the hands from exposure to blood and other bodily fluids.

68. Which type of PPE is designed to protect the eyes from splashes or sprays during a phlebotomy procedure?
a) Gloves
b) Goggles
c) Face shield
d) Mask

Answer: b) Goggles. Explanation: Goggles are used to protect the eyes from potential splashes or sprays of blood or other body fluids during procedures such as phlebotomy.

69. In addition to gloves, what other piece of PPE is typically used in most phlebotomy procedures?
a) Lab coat or gown
b) Respirator
c) Shoe covers
d) Ear plugs

Answer: a) Lab coat or gown. Explanation: A lab coat or gown is typically used in most phlebotomy procedures to protect the healthcare worker's clothing and skin from potential exposure to blood or other body fluids.

70. When should a face shield be used in addition to goggles during a phlebotomy procedure?
a) When the patient has a respiratory infection
b) When the procedure involves a large amount of blood
c) When the healthcare worker wears glasses
d) When the patient is uncooperative

Answer: a) When the patient has a respiratory infection. Explanation: A face shield should be used in addition to goggles when the patient has a respiratory infection to protect the healthcare worker from potential exposure to infectious droplets.

71. Which type of PPE should be used when there is a risk of airborne transmission of pathogens?
a) Gloves
b) Lab coat
c) Mask
d) Respirator

Answer: d) Respirator. Explanation: A respirator is a type of PPE that should be used when there is a risk of airborne transmission of pathogens. It provides a higher level of respiratory protection than a mask.

72. What type of mask should be used during a phlebotomy procedure on a patient with Tuberculosis?
a) Surgical mask
b) N95 respirator
c) Cloth mask
d) Face shield

Answer: b) N95 respirator. Explanation: An N95 respirator should be used when performing a phlebotomy procedure on a patient with Tuberculosis as it provides a higher level of respiratory protection and is designed to filter out airborne particles.

73. When should shoe covers be used as part of PPE in a phlebotomy setting?
a) When the floor is wet
b) When the procedure involves a large amount of blood
c) When the healthcare worker has open wounds on their feet
d) When the patient has a foot infection

Answer: b) When the procedure involves a large amount of blood. Explanation: Shoe covers can be used as part of PPE in a phlebotomy setting when the procedure involves a large amount of blood, which could potentially splatter on the floor.

74. What type of gloves should be used during a phlebotomy procedure on a patient with a known latex allergy?
a) Latex gloves
b) Vinyl gloves
c) Nitrile gloves
d) Leather gloves

Answer: c) Nitrile gloves. Explanation: Nitrile gloves should be used when performing a phlebotomy procedure on a patient with a known latex allergy. Nitrile is a synthetic material that does not contain latex and is safe for individuals with latex allergies.

75. Which piece of PPE is recommended for use when cleaning up a large blood spill?
a) Gloves
b) Goggles
c) Gown
d) All of the above

Answer: d) All of the above. Explanation: When cleaning up a large blood spill, it is recommended to use a full set of PPE including gloves, goggles, and a gown to protect against potential exposure to bloodborne pathogens.

76. In a phlebotomy setting, when should a healthcare worker change their gloves?
a) After every patient
b) Every hour
c) Every four patients
d) At the end of the shift

Answer: a) After every patient. Explanation: In a phlebotomy setting, gloves should be changed after every patient to prevent cross-contamination.

77. Which of the following can occur from improper use of gloves in a healthcare setting?
a) Cross-contamination
b) Physical injury
c) Allergic reactions
d) All of the above

Answer: d) All of the above. Explanation: Improper use of gloves can lead to cross-contamination between patients, physical injury if they fail during a procedure, and allergic reactions if the user or patient has a latex allergy.

78. What can be a consequence of not properly disposing of used Personal Protective Equipment (PPE)?
a) It can be reused safely
b) It can cause harm to the environment
c) It can be a source of infection spread
d) It can be a source of a fire hazard

Answer: c) It can be a source of infection spread. Explanation: If used PPE is not properly disposed of, it can be a source of infection spread. PPE can be contaminated with bodily fluids, and if not handled correctly post-use, it can contribute to the spread of infectious diseases.

79. Why is it important to change gloves between patients?
a) It is not necessary to change gloves between patients
b) To prevent the transfer of microorganisms from one patient to another
c) To prevent the gloves from tearing
d) To allow the healthcare worker's hands to breathe

Answer: b) To prevent the transfer of microorganisms from one patient to another. Explanation: Gloves can pick up microorganisms from one patient and can be transferred to another if not changed, leading to cross-contamination and potentially infection.

80. What can be a potential consequence of not properly fitting a face mask?
a) It can limit the healthcare worker's visibility
b) It can increase the risk of transmission of infectious diseases
c) It can cause skin irritation
d) All of the above

Answer: b) It can increase the risk of transmission of infectious diseases. Explanation: A face mask that does not fit properly can allow infectious particles to be inhaled or exhaled, increasing the risk of transmission of infectious diseases.

81. What potential hazard can occur from reusing disposable gloves?
a) They can become more comfortable to wear
b) They can break more easily, exposing the healthcare worker to infectious material
c) They can cause skin irritation
d) They can lose their color

Answer: b) They can break more easily, exposing the healthcare worker to infectious material.
Explanation: Reusing disposable gloves can cause them to degrade and become more susceptible to tearing or puncturing, which can expose the healthcare worker to potentially infectious material.

82. What can be a consequence of wearing Personal Protective Equipment (PPE) for a prolonged period?
a) It can cause heat stress and dehydration
b) It can enhance the healthcare worker's performance
c) It can increase the life span of the PPE
d) It can make the PPE more comfortable to wear

Answer: a) It can cause heat stress and dehydration. Explanation: Wearing PPE for a prolonged period can increase body temperature, potentially leading to heat stress and dehydration. This is particularly true for full-body PPE and in hot environments.

83. Why is it important to inspect PPE before use?
a) To ensure it fits properly
b) To ensure it is not damaged or contaminated
c) To ensure it is the correct PPE for the task
d) All of the above

Answer: d) All of the above. Explanation: Inspecting PPE before use is crucial to ensure that it fits correctly, is not damaged or contaminated, and is the correct PPE for the task at hand. Any of these issues could potentially lead to an increased risk of exposure to infectious material.

84. What hazard can occur from not properly removing gloves?
a) They can be reused safely
b) The healthcare worker can be exposed to infectious material
c) The healthcare worker's hands can become too dry
d) They can become more comfortable to wear

Answer: b) The healthcare worker can be exposed to infectious material. Explanation: If gloves are not properly removed, the healthcare worker's hands can come into contact with the outside of the gloves, which may be contaminated with infectious material.

85. What can be a potential consequence of not using Personal Protective Equipment (PPE)?
a) Increased comfort
b) Increased risk of infection transmission
c) Improved patient interaction
d) Reduced equipment costs

Answer: b) Increased risk of infection transmission. Explanation: PPE is a barrier between healthcare workers and potentially infectious material. Not using PPE can increase the risk of infection transmission to both the healthcare worker and the patient.

86. What should you do if a needlestick injury occurs during a phlebotomy procedure?
a) Continue with the procedure
b) Immediately wash the area with soap and water
c) Ignore it, the risk of infection is minimal
d) Apply an antiseptic and continue with the procedure

Answer: b) Immediately wash the area with soap and water. Explanation: If a needlestick injury occurs, you should immediately stop the procedure, remove your gloves, wash the affected area with soap and water, and report the incident. Immediate washing can help reduce the risk of infection.

87. After a needle has been used, it is appropriate to:
a) Recap the needle
b) Dispose of it in the regular trash
c) Dispose of it in a sharps container
d) Clean it for reuse

Answer: c) Dispose of it in a sharps container. Explanation: Used needles are considered biohazardous waste and should be disposed of in a puncture-proof sharps container to prevent needlestick injuries.

88. If a sharps container is full, what should you do?
a) Continue using it until there is no more room
b) Seal it and replace it with a new one
c) Dispose of it in the regular trash
d) Empty it and reuse it

Answer: b) Seal it and replace it with a new one. Explanation: When a sharps container is full, it should be sealed to prevent spills and replaced with a new one to avoid overfilling and potential needlestick injuries.

89. During a phlebotomy procedure, where should the sharps container be located?
a) In a cupboard away from the procedure area
b) Close to the healthcare worker performing the procedure
c) In a different room entirely
d) Anywhere, it doesn't matter

Answer: b) Close to the healthcare worker performing the procedure. Explanation: The sharps container should be within arm's reach of the healthcare worker performing the procedure. This minimizes the distance that the sharp has to be carried, reducing the risk of a needlestick injury.

90. What should you do if you drop a used needle on the floor?
a) Pick it up with your hands and dispose of it
b) Use a dustpan and brush to clean it up
c) Use a piece of paper or cardboard to pick it up
d) Leave it, it's too dangerous to pick up

Answer: c) Use a piece of paper or cardboard to pick it up. Explanation: If a used needle is dropped on the floor, it should not be picked up with bare hands. Using a piece of paper or cardboard can help prevent a needlestick injury. It should then be disposed of in a sharps container.

91. What should you do with a used needle immediately after withdrawing it from the patient?
a) Recap it
b) Place it on the tray next to the patient
c) Dispose of it in a sharps container
d) Hand it to a colleague for disposal

Answer: c) Dispose of it in a sharps container. Explanation: After withdrawing a used needle from a patient, it should immediately be disposed of in a sharps container to minimize the risk of a needlestick injury.

92. What should you do if the sharps container is not within reach during a phlebotomy procedure?
a) Leave the used needle on the tray and move it to the sharps container later
b) Hand the used needle to a colleague to dispose of
c) Recap the needle and place it aside for later disposal
d) Ask the patient to hold the needle while you get the sharps container

Answer: b) Hand the used needle to a colleague to dispose of.

93. What should a phlebotomist do immediately after using a needle?
a) Dispose it in the general waste bin
b) Place it on the tray for later disposal
c) Recap the needle
d) Dispose it in a puncture-resistant sharps container

Answer: d) Dispose it in a puncture-resistant sharps container. Explanation: Immediately after use, sharps such as needles should be placed in a designated, puncture-resistant sharps container to prevent needlestick injuries and potential disease transmission.

94. What is a critical consideration when selecting the location for a sharps container in a phlebotomy procedure?
a) It should be out of patients' sight
b) It should be in an easily accessible location
c) It should be near the floor
d) It should be behind the phlebotomist

Answer: b) It should be in an easily accessible location. Explanation: The sharps container should be located within arm's reach to allow for immediate disposal of sharps. This reduces the risk of accidental needlestick injuries.

95. How should sharps containers be disposed of when they become full?
a) They should be emptied into the general trash
b) They should be sealed and labeled, then picked up by a biomedical waste disposal company
c) They should be sealed and recycled
d) They should be washed and reused

Answer: b) They should be sealed and labeled, then picked up by a biomedical waste disposal company. Explanation: When a sharps container becomes full, it should be sealed and labeled for collection by a licensed biomedical waste disposal company. It's crucial to ensure these materials are disposed of properly to prevent harm and potential infection.

96. What is the purpose of the 'no recap' rule when dealing with needles?
a) To conserve resources
b) To speed up the procedure
c) To prevent needlestick injuries
d) To improve patient comfort

Answer: c) To prevent needlestick injuries. Explanation: The 'no recap' rule exists to prevent needlestick injuries that can occur when attempting to recap a used needle. These injuries can potentially transmit infectious diseases.

97. In the event of a needlestick injury, what is the first action to take?
a) Continue with the procedure
b) Wash the area with soap and water
c) Apply an adhesive bandage
d) Report to your supervisor

Answer: b) Wash the area with soap and water. Explanation: After a needlestick injury, it's important to immediately wash the affected area with soap and water to reduce the risk of infection. The injury should then be reported for further medical evaluation and treatment.

98. How should a phlebotomist handle a broken glass tube during a procedure?
a) Pick it up with their hands
b) Use a brush and dustpan or tongs
c) Sweep it under the counter
d) Leave it and continue with the procedure

Answer: b) Use a brush and dustpan or tongs. Explanation: If a glass tube breaks, it should be picked up using a mechanical tool like a brush and dustpan or tongs to prevent injuries. Never attempt to pick up broken glass with your hands, even when wearing gloves.

99. What should a phlebotomist do with a syringe after drawing blood?
a) Recap the needle and dispose of it in the sharps container
b) Remove the needle, recap it, then dispose of the syringe and needle separately
c) Immediately dispose of it in the sharps container without recapping
d) Reuse it for the next patient

Answer: c) Immediately dispose of it in the sharps container without recapping. Explanation: Following blood draw, the entire syringe should be immediately disposed of in the sharps container without recapping the needle.

100. What is the most common consequence of improper handling of sharps?
a) Misdiagnosis of patient's condition
b) Cross-contamination between samples
c) Needlestick injuries
d) Contamination of the work area

Answer: c) Needlestick injuries. Explanation: Needlestick injuries are the most common consequence of improper handling of sharps. They pose a serious risk to healthcare workers, as they can lead to the transmission of bloodborne pathogens.

101. Which of the following diseases can potentially be transmitted through needlestick injuries?
a) Tuberculosis
b) Influenza
c) Hepatitis B
d) Malaria

Answer: c) Hepatitis B. Explanation: Hepatitis B, along with Hepatitis C and HIV, are among the serious diseases that can potentially be transmitted through needlestick injuries due to the direct contact with infected blood.

102. What is the first step to mitigate the risk of needlestick injuries?
a) Using blunt needles
b) Double gloving
c) Using safety-engineered devices
d) Recapping needles

Answer: c) Using safety-engineered devices. Explanation: The first step to mitigating the risk of needlestick injuries is using safety-engineered devices, such as self-sheathing needles or retractable syringes. These devices have built-in safety control devices, such as a shield or a retractable needle, that can help prevent injuries.

103. How can the risk of needlestick injuries be reduced after using a sharp device?
a) Leaving the needle uncapped on the tray for later disposal
b) Recapping the needle before disposal
c) Immediately disposing of the used sharp in a designated sharps container
d) Cleaning the used sharp with disinfectant before disposal

Answer: c) Immediately disposing of the used sharp in a designated sharps container. Explanation: After using a sharp, it should be immediately disposed of in a designated sharps container to prevent needlestick injuries. This prevents accidental contact with the used sharp.

104. How can one reduce the risk of injuries when a sharps container is full?
a) By pushing down the sharps to make more room
b) By recapping the sharps before disposal
c) By sealing the sharps container and using a new one
d) By taking out some sharps and using a different container

Answer: c) By sealing the sharps container and using a new one. Explanation: When a sharps container is full, it should be sealed to prevent spillage or accidental stick injuries. A new container should then be used. Overfilling a sharps container increases the risk of accidental injuries.

105. What should you do if a needlestick injury occurs?
a) Continue with the procedure
b) Wash the area with soap and water, then report the injury
c) Apply a bandage and continue working
d) Ignore it if there's no visible blood

Answer: b) Wash the area with soap and water, then report the injury. Explanation: If a needlestick injury occurs, you should immediately wash the area with soap and water, then report the injury for medical follow-up and treatment as necessary.

106. What is an effective strategy for preventing needlestick injuries in a healthcare setting?
a) Using more personal protective equipment
b) Implementing a needlestick injury prevention program
c) Using less sharps in procedures
d) Recapping needles before disposal

Answer: b) Implementing a needlestick injury prevention program. Explanation: Implementing a comprehensive needlestick injury prevention program, which includes education, safer device selection, and consistent use of safe work practices, can significantly reduce the risk of needlestick injuries in a healthcare setting.

107. Which of the following is a safe work practice when handling sharps?
a) Recapping needles with two hands
b) Passing sharps hand-to-hand
c) Placing sharps on the counter for later disposal
d) Not bending or breaking needles before disposal

Answer: d) Not bending or breaking needles before disposal. Explanation: Bending or breaking needles can lead to accidental injuries. Sharps should be disposed of immediately in a designated sharps container without manipulating them.

108. Why is it important to report all needlestick injuries?
a) To ensure the individual gets appropriate post-exposure prophylaxis
b) To ensure the patient is notified of the injury
c) To allow the healthcare worker to take time off
d) To document the number of injuries in the facility

Answer: a) To ensure the individual gets appropriate post-exposure prophylaxis. Explanation: Reporting needlestick injuries is critical because it allows the healthcare worker to receive immediate medical attention, including post-exposure prophylaxis for HIV, hepatitis B, or hepatitis C if required.

109. In addition to the use of safety-engineered devices, what else can help prevent needlestick injuries?
a) Routine recapping of needles
b) Using sharps only when necessary
c) Ignoring the 'no-pass' policy for sharps
d) Overfilling sharps containers

Answer: b) Using sharps only when necessary. Explanation: Limiting the use of sharps only to procedures where they are absolutely necessary is another strategy to prevent needlestick injuries. The fewer the sharps in use, the lower the risk of injuries.

110. After a blood collection procedure, where should the used sharps be placed?
a) In the regular trash can
b) In the recycling bin
c) Directly in the sink for washing
d) In a puncture-proof sharps container

Answer: d) In a puncture-proof sharps container. Explanation: Used sharps should be immediately placed in a puncture-proof sharps container. This reduces the risk of needlestick injuries and environmental contamination.

111. What is the correct way to handle a used needle immediately after blood collection?
a) Recap the needle and set it aside for later disposal
b) Remove the needle from the syringe and place it in the sharps container
c) With one hand, immediately place the needle and syringe into the sharps container
d) Clean the needle with alcohol before disposing of it in the sharps container

Answer: c) With one hand, immediately place the needle and syringe into the sharps container. Explanation: The entire needle and syringe unit should be disposed of as one item in the sharps container immediately after use. Recapping, removing, or cleaning the needle increases the risk of a needlestick injury.

112. What should be done if the sharps container is full?
a) Push down the sharps to make more room
b) Add a bag liner and continue using it
c) Seal it and replace it with a new container
d) Take it outside for disposal

Answer: c) Seal it and replace it with a new container. Explanation: A full sharps container should be sealed and replaced with a new container. Overfilling a sharps container increases the risk of a needlestick injury.

113. What should not be done with a used needle before placing it in a sharps container?
a) Cleaning it
b) Recapping it
c) Breaking it
d) All of the above

Answer: d) All of the above. Explanation: Used needles should not be recapped, bent, broken, or cleaned. These actions increase the risk of a needlestick injury.

114. Why is it necessary to avoid touching the outside of the sharps container?
a) It may have blood or other bodily fluids on it
b) It is not necessary to avoid touching the outside
c) It could cause the container to fall over
d) It could cause a needlestick injury

Answer: a) It may have blood or other bodily fluids on it. Explanation: The outside of a sharps container could be contaminated with blood or other bodily fluids, so it's important to avoid touching it with bare hands.

115. Which of the following is an important part of safe sharps disposal?
a) Washing used sharps before disposal
b) Leaving the sharps container open after use
c) Regularly checking the fill level of sharps containers
d) Using sharps containers that are easily penetrable

Answer: c) Regularly checking the fill level of sharps containers. Explanation: Regularly checking the fill level of sharps containers is crucial. This prevents overfilling, which can lead to spills or needlestick injuries.

116. Which of the following is a safe practice for sharps disposal?
a) Placing the sharps container in an easily accessible location
b) Positioning the sharps container at a low level where it can be easily reached
c) Filling the sharps container to the top before replacing it
d) Emptying the sharps container into a larger bin when it is full

Answer: a) Placing the sharps container in an easily accessible location. Explanation: Sharps containers should be easily accessible and located as close as possible to the point of use. This reduces the risk of accidents when disposing of sharps.

117. When should the sharps container be replaced?
a) When it is three-quarters full
b) When it is completely full
c) When it is half full
d) At the end of the day, regardless of how full it is

Answer: a) When it is three-quarters full. Explanation: Sharps containers should be replaced when they are about three-quarters full to prevent overfilling and potential spills or needlestick injuries.

118. What should be done if a needlestick injury occurs during the disposal process?
a) Clean the wound, report the incident, and seek medical attention
b) Continue working and deal with the injury later
c) Rinse the wound with water only
d) Ignore the injury as it's part of the job risk

Answer: a) Clean the wound, report the incident, and seek medical attention. Explanation: If a needlestick or sharps injury occurs, it's important to immediately clean the wound, report the incident to the appropriate person, and seek medical attention. This is important for early treatment and prevention of infection.

119. What should be done with the sharps container once it is three-quarters full?
a) It should be opened and the contents sorted for recycling
b) It should be sealed and replaced with a new container
c) It should be emptied into a larger container for disposal
d) It should be left until it is completely full

Answer: b) It should be sealed and replaced with a new container. Explanation: Once a sharps container is three-quarters full, it should be sealed to prevent spills or accidents. It should then be replaced with a new container for future sharps disposal.

120. How can the use of Personal Protective Equipment (PPE) contribute to reducing Healthcare-Associated Infections (HAIs)?
a) By protecting the patient from infections the healthcare worker might be carrying
b) By creating a physical barrier between pathogens and the healthcare worker
c) By preventing the spread of pathogens in the healthcare setting
d) All of the above

Answer: d) All of the above. Explanation: PPE creates a physical barrier between the healthcare worker and potential pathogens, protecting both parties. It also prevents the spread of these pathogens within the healthcare setting, reducing the likelihood of HAIs.

121. What role does hand hygiene play in reducing HAIs?
a) Hand hygiene is not related to HAIs
b) Hand hygiene can reduce the spread of pathogens from patient to patient
c) Hand hygiene can protect the healthcare worker from infections
d) Both b and c

Answer: d) Both b and c. Explanation: Hand hygiene is a crucial step in preventing the spread of infections in a healthcare setting. It can protect the healthcare worker and also prevent the spread of pathogens from one patient to another.

122. How can proper sharps disposal contribute to reducing HAIs?
a) It prevents the spread of infections through accidental pricks
b) It prevents the re-use of sharps
c) It keeps the environment clean
d) All of the above

Answer: d) All of the above. Explanation: Proper sharps disposal can prevent accidental pricks that can lead to the spread of infections. It also ensures that sharps are not re-used and contributes to maintaining a clean environment, reducing the risk of HAIs.

123. What is the significance of patient isolation in reducing HAIs?
a) It doesn't play a role in reducing HAIs
b) It prevents the spread of infection from the isolated patient to others
c) It protects the isolated patient from contracting other infections
d) Both b and c

Answer: d) Both b and c. Explanation: Patient isolation is a crucial strategy in preventing the spread of infections within a healthcare setting. It protects other patients from the isolated patient's infection and also protects the isolated patient from contracting other infections.

124. How does regular cleaning and disinfection of the healthcare environment contribute to reducing HAIs?
a) It removes any potential pathogens present in the environment
b) It reduces the risk of transmission of infections through contact with surfaces
c) It helps maintain a healthy environment for both patients and healthcare workers
d) All of the above

Answer: d) All of the above. Explanation: Regular cleaning and disinfection removes potential pathogens from the healthcare environment and reduces the risk of transmission of infections through contact with surfaces. It helps in maintaining a healthy environment for both patients and healthcare workers.

125. How does following the principles of aseptic technique contribute to reducing HAIs?
a) By preventing contamination of sterile areas and items
b) By reducing the risk of infections following surgical procedures
c) By ensuring that pathogens are not introduced into vulnerable body sites
d) All of the above

Answer: d) All of the above. Explanation: The principles of aseptic technique prevent contamination of sterile areas and items, reduce the risk of post-surgical infections, and ensure that pathogens are not introduced into vulnerable body sites. This greatly contributes to reducing HAIs.

126. Why is vaccination of healthcare workers important in the prevention of HAIs?
a) Vaccinated healthcare workers cannot transmit diseases to patients
b) Vaccination doesn't affect the rate of HAIs
c) Vaccination protects healthcare workers from diseases that can be passed on to patients
d) Vaccination allows healthcare workers to work without using PPE

Answer: c) Vaccination protects healthcare workers from diseases that can be passed on to patients.
Explanation: Vaccination of healthcare workers is important as it reduces their susceptibility to certain diseases, which can be passed on to patients if the healthcare worker becomes infected.

127. How can correct and consistent use of PPE reduce HAIs?
a) By minimizing direct contact with infectious agents
b) By preventing the spread of infectious agents from healthcare workers to patients
c) By protecting healthcare workers from potential infections
d) All of the above

Answer: d) All of the above. Explanation: Correct and consistent use of PPE can minimize direct contact with infectious agents, prevent the spread of infectious agents from healthcare workers to patients, and protect healthcare workers from potential infections.

128. Why is proper ventilation important in preventing HAIs?
a) Proper ventilation doesn't play a role in preventing HAIs
b) Proper ventilation can prevent the spread of airborne pathogens
c) Proper ventilation can keep the healthcare environment clean
d) Both b and c

Answer: b) Proper ventilation can prevent the spread of airborne pathogens. Explanation: Good ventilation in healthcare settings is critical as it helps prevent the spread of airborne pathogens that could cause HAIs.

129. How can safety and infection control procedures reduce the incidence of multi-drug resistant infections in healthcare settings?
a) By preventing the spread of pathogens that may develop resistance
b) By reducing the need for excessive use of antibiotics, which can lead to resistance
c) By ensuring that all infections are treated promptly and correctly
d) All of the above

Answer: d) All of the above. Explanation: Safety and infection control procedures can help prevent the spread of pathogens that may develop resistance, reduce the need for excessive use of antibiotics, and ensure that infections are treated promptly and correctly, all of which can help reduce the incidence of multi-drug resistant infections.

130. What strategy can help ensure staff are following safety and infection control procedures?
a) Ignoring minor breaches in protocol
b) Regular audits and spot checks
c) Relying on staff to self-regulate
d) Providing less training to experienced staff

Answer: b) Regular audits and spot checks. Explanation: Regular audits and spot checks are effective ways to ensure that staff are consistently following safety and infection control procedures. These checks can identify breaches in protocol that need to be corrected.

131. What role does training play in ensuring compliance with safety and infection control procedures?
a) Training is not important as long as staff are experienced
b) Training helps staff understand the importance of the procedures
c) Training is only necessary for new staff
d) Training can make staff too cautious

Answer: b) Training helps staff understand the importance of the procedures. Explanation: Training is essential to ensure that all staff, regardless of their level of experience, understand the importance of safety and infection control procedures and know how to apply them correctly.

132. What is the importance of clear, written guidelines in ensuring compliance with safety and infection control procedures?
a) Written guidelines are unnecessary
b) They provide a reference for staff to ensure they are following procedures correctly
c) They make it easier to blame staff for mistakes
d) They are less important than verbal instructions

Answer: b) They provide a reference for staff to ensure they are following procedures correctly. Explanation: Clear, written guidelines are important as they provide a reference that staff can use to ensure they are following safety and infection control procedures correctly.

133. How can management encourage compliance with safety and infection control procedures?
a) By ignoring minor breaches in protocol
b) By setting an example and following the procedures themselves
c) By only enforcing the rules when regulators are present
d) By relying on staff to self-regulate

Answer: b) By setting an example and following the procedures themselves. Explanation: Management can encourage compliance by setting an example and demonstrating commitment to safety and infection control procedures. This can motivate staff to do the same.

134. What is the role of continuous improvement in ensuring compliance with safety and infection control procedures?
a) Continuous improvement is less important than strict enforcement
b) Continuous improvement allows for adaptation and improvement of procedures based on feedback and new information
c) Continuous improvement should only be considered after a breach in protocol
d) Continuous improvement is not related to compliance with safety and infection control procedures

Answer: b) Continuous improvement allows for adaptation and improvement of procedures based on feedback and new information. Explanation: Continuous improvement can enhance compliance by allowing for procedures to be regularly reviewed and updated based on feedback and new information. This keeps procedures relevant and effective.

135. How can feedback from staff contribute to compliance with safety and infection control procedures?
a) Staff feedback is not important
b) Staff feedback can identify areas where procedures are not being followed and suggest improvements
c) Staff feedback should only be considered after a breach in protocol
d) Staff feedback can make procedures too complex

Answer: b) Staff feedback can identify areas where procedures are not being followed and suggest improvements. Explanation: Staff feedback is valuable as it can identify areas of non-compliance and suggest possible improvements to the procedures, enhancing their effectiveness and ensuring better compliance.

136. What is the role of equipment maintenance in ensuring compliance with safety and infection control procedures?
a) Equipment maintenance is unrelated to compliance with safety and infection control procedures
b) Proper equipment maintenance ensures that safety and infection control procedures can be carried out effectively
c) Equipment maintenance should only be considered after a breach in protocol
d) Regular equipment maintenance makes procedures too complex

Answer: b) Proper equipment maintenance ensures that safety and infection control procedures can be carried out effectively. Explanation: Regular and proper equipment maintenance is necessary to ensure that safety and infection control procedures can be carried out effectively.

137. How can management handle non-compliance with safety and infection control procedures?
a) Ignore it if it's a minor breach
b) Provide constructive feedback and retrain if necessary
c) Punish the staff member involved harshly
d) Cover it up to protect the reputation of the facility

Answer: b) Provide constructive feedback and retrain if necessary. Explanation: When non-compliance is identified, management should provide constructive feedback to the staff member involved and retrain them if necessary, to ensure they understand the importance of compliance and how to follow the procedures correctly.

138. Why is it important to have a system for reporting and investigating breaches in safety and infection control procedures?
a) It's not important to investigate breaches
b) It allows for identification of areas for improvement and prevention of future breaches
c) It allows for punishment of non-compliant staff
d) It's only important if a patient was harmed

Answer: b) It allows for identification of areas for improvement and prevention of future breaches. Explanation: Having a system for reporting and investigating breaches is important as it can help identify areas for improvement and prevent similar breaches in the future.

139. How can periodic review and updating of safety and infection control procedures contribute to compliance?
a) They make the procedures too complex for staff to follow
b) They ensure the procedures remain relevant and effective
c) They are not necessary if the procedures were well-designed initially
d) They should only be done after a serious breach in protocol

Answer: b) They ensure the procedures remain relevant and effective. Explanation: Periodic review and updating of safety and infection control procedures help ensure they remain relevant and effective, which can contribute to better compliance. This process takes into account new research, changes in practices, and feedback from staff.

140. What could potentially happen if a phlebotomist doesn't change gloves between patients?
a) Nothing, as long as their hands appear clean
b) It can lead to the transmission of infections between patients
c) Patients might feel uncomfortable
d) The gloves might become uncomfortable to wear

Answer: b) It can lead to the transmission of infections between patients. Explanation: If a phlebotomist doesn't change gloves between patients, they can carry pathogens from one patient to another, potentially causing infections. Even if gloves appear clean, they can harbor microscopic pathogens.

141. What could be the outcome if sharps are not disposed of properly in a phlebotomy setting?
a) Nothing, as long as they are kept out of patients' sight
b) It can increase the risk of needlestick injuries
c) It can lead to a cluttered workspace
d) Sharps can lose their sharpness

Answer: b) It can increase the risk of needlestick injuries. Explanation: Improper disposal of sharps can lead to needlestick injuries, which can transmit infections such as HIV, Hepatitis B and C.

142. What is a potential consequence if a phlebotomist doesn't use a safety-engineered needle for a blood draw?
a) It might take longer to draw blood
b) There's an increased risk of a needlestick injury after the procedure
c) The needle might break in the patient's vein
d) The blood might clot in the needle

Answer: b) There's an increased risk of a needlestick injury after the procedure. Explanation: Safety-engineered needles are designed to prevent needlestick injuries after the procedure. If they're not used, the risk of such injuries increases.

143. What can result from a phlebotomist not following the correct order of draw?
a) There might be more discomfort for the patient
b) It could lead to cross-contamination of additives between tubes
c) The phlebotomist might get confused
d) The tubes might break

Answer: b) It could lead to cross-contamination of additives between tubes. Explanation: The correct order of draw prevents the cross-contamination of additives between tubes, which could affect the accuracy of test results.

144. What might happen if a phlebotomist doesn't sanitize their hands before putting on gloves?
a) The gloves might tear
b) There might be discomfort due to sweating
c) Pathogens on the hand can be transferred to the inside of the glove
d) The gloves might not fit properly

Answer: c) Pathogens on the hand can be transferred to the inside of the glove. Explanation: If a phlebotomist doesn't sanitize their hands before putting on gloves, any pathogens present on the hands can be transferred to the inside of the gloves and potentially cause infection.

145. What is a possible consequence if a phlebotomist reuses a tourniquet on different patients without cleaning it?
a) The tourniquet might lose elasticity
b) It can lead to the spread of infections between patients
c) Patients might find it uncomfortable
d) The tourniquet might break

Answer: b) It can lead to the spread of infections between patients. Explanation: A tourniquet can come into contact with a patient's skin and body fluids. If it's reused without being cleaned, it can spread pathogens between patients.

146. What could be the outcome if a phlebotomist does not properly label a blood sample?
a) The sample might be discarded
b) The lab might process the sample for the wrong test
c) The wrong patient might get the results
d) All of the above

Answer: d) All of the above. Explanation: Proper labeling of blood samples is crucial to ensure they are correctly processed and the results are delivered to the right patient. If a sample is not properly labeled, it could be discarded, processed for the wrong test, or the results could be sent to the wrong patient.

147. What could be a consequence of not adhering to patient identification procedures during phlebotomy?
a) There is a chance of a misidentification error, potentially leading to incorrect treatment
b) The phlebotomist might draw blood from the wrong vein
c) The patient might feel uncomfortable
d) It can take longer to draw blood

Answer: a) There is a chance of a misidentification error, potentially leading to incorrect treatment. Explanation: Correct patient identification is crucial in phlebotomy to prevent misidentification errors, which can have serious consequences, including incorrect treatment.

148. What is the potential risk if a phlebotomist does not adhere to the recommended angle of needle insertion during venipuncture?
a) The patient might feel more pain
b) It can lead to unsuccessful venipuncture or injury to the patient
c) The needle might break
d) The procedure might take longer

Answer: b) It can lead to unsuccessful venipuncture or injury to the patient. Explanation: The recommended angle of needle insertion is crucial for successful venipuncture and to avoid injury to the patient.

149. What could happen if a phlebotomist does not release the tourniquet within the recommended time during a blood draw?
a) The patient might feel discomfort
b) It can lead to hemoconcentration, affecting test results
c) The tourniquet might break
d) The patient might faint

Answer: b) It can lead to hemoconcentration, affecting test results. Explanation: If the tourniquet is not released within the recommended time, it can lead to hemoconcentration, which is an increase in the concentration of larger molecules and cells in the blood. This can affect the accuracy of certain blood tests.

150. Why are safety and infection control procedures important in phlebotomy?
a) They help in organizing the work efficiently
b) They ensure the phlebotomist looks professional
c) They protect both the patient and the healthcare provider from potential infection
d) They help the phlebotomist to draw blood faster

Answer: c) They protect both the patient and the healthcare provider from potential infection. Explanation: Safety and infection control procedures are designed to prevent the spread of infection, protecting both patients and healthcare providers.

151 Why is it crucial to use a new pair of gloves for each patient in phlebotomy?
a) Because it makes the patient feel more comfortable
b) Because it helps the phlebotomist maintain a good grip on the equipment
c) To prevent the transmission of pathogens from one patient to another
d) To prevent the gloves from tearing

Answer: c) To prevent the transmission of pathogens from one patient to another. Explanation: Gloves can harbor pathogens which can be transferred from one patient to another, potentially causing infections.

152. Why is it important to disinfect the venipuncture site before drawing blood?
a) To make sure the area looks clean
b) To make the procedure less painful for the patient
c) To kill any potential pathogens on the skin that could enter the blood sample
d) To help the needle penetrate the skin more easily

Answer: c) To kill any potential pathogens on the skin that could enter the blood sample. Explanation: Disinfecting the venipuncture site kills any potential pathogens on the skin that could contaminate the blood sample or enter the patient's bloodstream during the procedure.

153. Why is following the correct order of draw essential in phlebotomy?
a) To make the procedure faster
b) To prevent cross-contamination of additives between tubes
c) To ensure the tubes are filled in the order they are arranged on the tray
d) To make the procedure less painful for the patient

Answer: b) To prevent cross-contamination of additives between tubes. Explanation: The correct order of draw prevents cross-contamination of additives between tubes, which could interfere with test results.

154. Why should sharps be disposed of in a designated sharps container immediately after use?
a) To keep the workspace tidy
b) To make it easier to count the number of sharps used
c) To prevent accidental needlestick injuries
d) To ensure the sharps do not lose their sharpness

Answer: c) To prevent accidental needlestick injuries. Explanation: Disposing of sharps immediately after use in a designated sharps container can prevent accidental needlestick injuries, which pose a risk of transmitting bloodborne pathogens.

155. What is the significance of patient identification in phlebotomy safety and infection control procedures?
a) To ensure the patient is comfortable with the phlebotomist
b) To prevent errors such as collecting specimens from the wrong patient or attributing results to the wrong patient
c) To make sure the phlebotomist remembers the patient's name
d) To ensure the phlebotomist collects the right amount of blood

Answer: b) To prevent errors such as collecting specimens from the wrong patient or attributing results to the wrong patient. Explanation: Correct patient identification is crucial in preventing dangerous errors such as collecting specimens from the wrong patient or attributing lab results to the wrong patient.

156. Why is proper hand hygiene important in phlebotomy safety and infection control procedures?
a) To prevent the transmission of pathogens
b) To ensure the phlebotomist's hands are comfortable during the procedure
c) To ensure the patient feels comfortable with the phlebotomist touching them
d) To prevent the phlebotomist's hands from becoming dry

Answer: a) To prevent the transmission of pathogens. Explanation: Proper hand hygiene is a simple yet crucial step in preventing the transmission of pathogens, thus protecting both the patient and the healthcare provider.

157. What is the significance of properly cleaning and disinfecting phlebotomy equipment?
a) To ensure the equipment looks presentable
b) To prevent the spread of pathogens and reduce the risk of healthcare-associated infections
c) To make the equipment last longer
d) To ensure the equipment works efficiently

Answer: b) To prevent the spread of pathogens and reduce the risk of healthcare-associated infections. Explanation: Properly cleaning and disinfecting phlebotomy equipment is important to prevent the spread of pathogens and thereby reduce the risk of healthcare-associated infections.

158. What is the potential consequence of not following safety and infection control procedures in phlebotomy?
a) The phlebotomist might feel less confident
b) The procedure might take longer
c) It can lead to the spread of infections, cause harm to patients and healthcare providers, and potentially have legal implications
d) The phlebotomist might not be able to draw blood successfully

Answer: c) It can lead to the spread of infections, cause harm to patients and healthcare providers, and potentially have legal implications. Explanation: Not following safety and infection control procedures in phlebotomy can have serious consequences, including the spread of infections, harm to patients and healthcare providers, and potentially even legal implications.

159. What role does personal protective equipment (PPE) play in safety and infection control procedures in phlebotomy?
a) It helps the phlebotomist feel more comfortable during the procedure
b) It protects the phlebotomist and the patient from potential exposure to bloodborne pathogens
c) It ensures the phlebotomist looks professional
d) It makes the procedure less painful for the patient

Answer: b) It protects the phlebotomist and the patient from potential exposure to bloodborne pathogens. Explanation: Personal protective equipment (PPE) is a critical part of safety and infection control procedures in phlebotomy. It protects both the phlebotomist and the patient from potential exposure to bloodborne pathogens.

160. What is the primary purpose of Standard Precautions in the healthcare setting?
a) To protect healthcare workers from patients
b) To decrease the number of patients a healthcare worker sees in a day
c) To protect both healthcare workers and patients from potential infection
d) To ensure healthcare workers are comfortable while working

Answer: c) To protect both healthcare workers and patients from potential infection. Explanation: Standard Precautions are designed to protect healthcare workers and patients alike by minimizing the risk of transmitting infections.

161. Which of the following practices is NOT included in the Standard Precautions?
a) Disinfecting hands before and after every patient contact
b) Wearing personal protective equipment (PPE) only when dealing with known infectious patients
c) Proper handling and disposal of sharps
d) Using a new pair of gloves for every patient

Answer: b) Wearing personal protective equipment (PPE) only when dealing with known infectious patients. Explanation: Standard Precautions apply to all patients, regardless of their infection status. PPE should be used as needed, based on the nature of the potential exposure.

162. What does the concept of "treat all blood, body fluids, secretions, and excretions as if they were infectious" refer to in Standard Precautions?
a) Infection control
b) PPE use
c) Hand hygiene
d) Source isolation

Answer: a) Infection control. Explanation: This concept is central to infection control as part of Standard Precautions, emphasizing that all bodily substances could potentially harbor infectious agents, regardless of the known presence of infectious disease.

163. Why is hand hygiene a critical aspect of Standard Precautions?
a) Because it's an easy and effective way to prevent the spread of pathogens
b) Because it helps healthcare workers stay clean
c) Because it's a regulatory requirement
d) Because it keeps patients comfortable

Answer: a) Because it's an easy and effective way to prevent the spread of pathogens. Explanation: Hand hygiene is one of the simplest and most effective ways to prevent the spread of pathogens, making it a crucial part of Standard Precautions.

164. How are respiratory hygiene and cough etiquette part of Standard Precautions?
a) They ensure healthcare workers don't catch colds
b) They prevent the spread of airborne and droplet-transmitted infections
c) They make patients feel comfortable
d) They prevent healthcare workers from coughing during procedures

Answer: b) They prevent the spread of airborne and droplet-transmitted infections. Explanation: Respiratory hygiene and cough etiquette are integral to Standard Precautions because they help to prevent the spread of airborne and droplet-transmitted infections.

165. Why is it important to properly clean and disinfect surfaces as part of Standard Precautions?
a) It makes the healthcare setting look more professional
b) It helps to prevent the spread of infections by eliminating pathogens from surfaces
c) It helps healthcare workers feel more comfortable
d) It ensures healthcare workers are busy

Answer: b) It helps to prevent the spread of infections by eliminating pathogens from surfaces. Explanation: Proper cleaning and disinfection of surfaces as part of Standard Precautions helps to minimize the risk of pathogens being transmitted from surfaces to individuals.

166. How does proper waste disposal contribute to Standard Precautions?
a) It helps to keep the healthcare setting tidy
b) It prevents the spread of infection by properly disposing of potentially contaminated materials
c) It ensures the waste bins don't overflow
d) It helps healthcare workers stay organized

Answer: b) It prevents the spread of infection by properly disposing of potentially contaminated materials. Explanation: Proper waste disposal is a key aspect of Standard Precautions, as it helps prevent the spread of infections by ensuring that potentially contaminated materials are disposed of appropriately.

167. Why are Standard Precautions considered the foundation of infection control in healthcare settings?
a) They are easy to implement
b) They are cost-effective
c) They provide a broad level of protection against the spread of pathogens in healthcare settings
d) They help healthcare workers feel more comfortable

Answer: c) They provide a broad level of protection against the spread of pathogens in healthcare settings. Explanation: Standard Precautions provide a comprehensive strategy for the prevention and control of infection in healthcare settings, making them the cornerstone of infection control.

168. Who should follow Standard Precautions in the healthcare setting?
a) Only doctors and nurses
b) Only healthcare workers dealing with known infectious patients
c) Only the infection control team
d) All healthcare workers, regardless of their role or the patients they care for

Answer: d) All healthcare workers, regardless of their role or the patients they care for. Explanation: Standard Precautions apply to all healthcare workers, regardless of their role or the type of patient they are caring for, because these precautions are designed to protect against the spread of infections from any potential source.

169. How do Standard Precautions help to protect patients in healthcare settings?
a) They ensure patients are comfortable during procedures
b) They reduce the risk of healthcare-associated infections
c) They ensure patients are cared for by healthy healthcare workers
d) They ensure patients receive care in a clean environment

Answer: b) They reduce the risk of healthcare-associated infections. Explanation: By implementing Standard Precautions, healthcare workers can significantly reduce the risk of healthcare-associated infections, thereby protecting the health and safety of patients.

170. At her healthcare facility, Nurse Maria sees a colleague leaving the patient's room without removing his gloves and gown. What is Maria's best course of action?
a) Ignore it and continue her work.
b) Report the colleague to their supervisor.
c) Educate the colleague about proper PPE disposal.
d) Take a photo for evidence.

Answer: c) Educate the colleague about proper PPE disposal. Explanation: Proper PPE disposal is a crucial part of infection control and safety measures. It's vital to remind and educate colleagues about it whenever necessary to maintain a safe healthcare environment.

171. During an emergency evacuation at a hospital, a staff member was spotted running towards the exit without assisting patients. What could have been done to avoid such behavior?
a) Punishment for non-compliance should have been communicated beforehand.
b) Regular emergency evacuation drills and training should have been conducted.
c) Security personnel should have stopped the staff member.
d) A lockdown should have been initiated.

Answer: b) Regular emergency evacuation drills and training should have been conducted. Explanation: Regular training ensures all staff know their responsibilities during an emergency, promoting safety and compliance.

172. Phlebotomist John noticed a minor cut on his finger after collecting a blood sample. What should John do next?
a) Wash his hands, apply antiseptic and bandage, then report the incident.
b) Continue with his work as it's just a minor cut.
c) Take a break.
d) Report to his supervisor and request for a day off.

Answer: a) Wash his hands, apply antiseptic and bandage, then report the incident. Explanation: Immediate care should be given to prevent infection. After caring for the wound, the incident should be reported as per the protocol.

173. During a surprise safety inspection, a fire extinguisher was found blocked by a cart in the hallway. Who is responsible for this violation?
a) The last person who used the cart.
b) The safety inspection team.
c) Everyone, as all staff share responsibility for safety.
d) The person who noticed but didn't rectify the situation.

Answer: c) Everyone, as all staff share responsibility for safety. Explanation: Safety in the healthcare environment is a collective responsibility. All staff members should ensure that safety equipment like fire extinguishers are accessible at all times.

174. Lab technician Sam noticed a sharps container is three-quarters full. What should Sam do?
a) Continue using it until it's completely full.
b) Ignore it as it's not his responsibility.
c) Replace the container and properly dispose of the nearly full one.
d) Report to his supervisor and wait for further instructions.

Answer: c) Replace the container and properly dispose of the nearly full one. Explanation: A sharps container should be replaced when it is three-quarters full to prevent accidental needlestick injuries and potential cross-contamination.

175. During a flu outbreak in a nursing home, some staff members were found not to have received their flu shots. How could the management ensure better compliance in the future?
a) Make vaccination a condition of employment.
b) Impose fines on unvaccinated staff.
c) Hold regular health and safety education sessions.
d) Exclude unvaccinated staff from work during outbreaks.

Answer: c) Hold regular health and safety education sessions. Explanation: Regular education sessions can help staff understand the importance of vaccinations in preventing the spread of diseases, leading to better compliance.

176. An intern was spotted wearing gloves while typing on a computer keyboard. What is wrong with this scenario?
a) The intern is wasting PPE.
b) The gloves could contaminate the keyboard.
c) The intern should be wearing additional PPE.
d) The intern should have asked for permission before using the computer.

Answer: b) The gloves could contaminate the keyboard. Explanation: Wearing gloves while typing could lead to cross-contamination. It's important to remove gloves and sanitize hands before touching non-clinical items.

177. In a training session, an experienced nurse mentioned to new hires that she occasionally ignores certain safety protocols because they take too much time. What should be done about this?
a) Report the nurse for non-compliance.
b) Ignore the comment as she's experienced.
c) Have a discussion about the importance of safety protocols.
d) Give her a promotion for efficiency.

Answer: c) Have a discussion about the importance of safety protocols. Explanation: Everyone must adhere to safety protocols, irrespective of their experience. Discussing this can help reinforce the importance of safety and compliance.

178. A patient's relative was observed moving around the ICU without a visitor's badge. How could this security breach be prevented in the future?
a) Install security cameras.
b) Increase the number of security personnel.
c) Restrict visiting hours.
d) Improve visitor check-in procedures.

Answer: d) Improve visitor check-in procedures. Explanation: Efficient check-in procedures can help monitor visitors and ensure they are correctly identified, minimizing the chance of unauthorized access.

179. The safety officer noticed that the records of the fire safety drills conducted in the past year were incomplete. What would be an appropriate response?
a) Ignore it as fire safety drills are a formality.
b) Conduct a surprise fire drill.
c) Update and complete the records immediately.
d) Conduct a meeting to discuss the importance of record keeping.

Answer: d) Conduct a meeting to discuss the importance of record keeping. Explanation: Incomplete records could imply non-compliance or lack of importance given to safety drills. A meeting to discuss the importance of accurate record keeping can help reinforce the importance of compliance.

180. At what point should a sharps container be replaced?
a) When it is one-third full.
b) When it is half full.
c) When it is three-quarters full.
d) When it is completely full.

Answer: c) When it is three-quarters full. Explanation: Sharps containers should be replaced when they are about three-quarters full to prevent injury and potential cross-contamination.

181. What is a crucial step to take after a sharps injury occurs?
a) Panic and inform everyone in the vicinity.
b) Rinse the area with warm water and soap, then report the injury.
c) Ignore it if it's a minor cut.
d) Remove gloves and continue work.

Answer: b) Rinse the area with warm water and soap, then report the injury. Explanation: Immediate care should be given to the wound and the incident should be reported as per the protocol for managing sharps injuries.

182. Where should used needles be disposed of?
a) A general waste bin.
b) A recycling bin.
c) A sharps container.
d) A special bag provided by the hospital.

Answer: c) A sharps container. Explanation: Used needles and other sharp objects should be disposed of in a designated sharps container to prevent accidental injury and contamination.

183. Should needles be recapped after use?
a) Yes, always.
b) No, never.
c) Yes, but only with a one-handed technique.
d) Yes, but only if there is no sharps container available.

Answer: b) No, never. Explanation: Recapping needles can lead to accidental needlestick injuries. Needles should be immediately placed in a sharps container after use.

184. If a sharps container is not immediately available, what should be done with the used sharps?
a) Leave them on a table.
b) Put them in a plastic bag.
c) Keep them with you until a sharps container is found.
d) Recap them and put them in a safe place.

Answer: c) Keep them with you until a sharps container is found. Explanation: Used sharps should never be left unattended. If a sharps container is not immediately available, the safest option is to keep the sharps with you until one can be located.

185. Who is responsible for the proper disposal of sharps?
a) The person who used the sharps.
b) The custodial staff.
c) The nurse in charge.
d) The hospital administration.

Answer: a) The person who used the sharps. Explanation: The person who uses the sharps is responsible for their safe disposal. This helps ensure safety and accountability in the healthcare setting.

186. What should be done if a sharps container is found to be overfilled?
a) Add more sharps to it anyway.
b) Close it and leave it for someone else to deal with.
c) Take some sharps out to make more room.
d) Secure it, label it, and replace it with a new container.

Answer: d) Secure it, label it, and replace it with a new container. Explanation: If a sharps container is overfilled, it should be securely closed, properly labelled, and replaced with a new container. Overfilled sharps containers can be hazardous.

187. What PPE should be worn when handling sharps?
a) Gloves only.
b) Face shield and gloves.
c) Gloves and a gown.
d) Gloves, gown, and goggles or a face shield.

Answer: d) Gloves, gown, and goggles or a face shield. Explanation: Proper PPE, including gloves, gown, and goggles or a face shield, should be worn when handling sharps to reduce the risk of exposure to bloodborne pathogens.

188. If a sharps container is accidentally knocked over, what should be done?
a) Quickly pick up the sharps and put them back in the container.
b) Leave the room and alert a supervisor.
c) Use tongs or forceps to pick up the sharps, wearing appropriate PPE.
d) Kick the sharps to the side to clear a path.

Answer: c) Use tongs or forceps to pick up the sharps, wearing appropriate PPE. Explanation: If a sharps container is knocked over, it's important to maintain safety. Sharps should be picked up with tongs or forceps while wearing appropriate PPE, to prevent accidental injury.

189. What is the primary reason for safe handling and disposal of sharps?
a) To reduce the risk of needlestick injuries.
b) To maintain a clean environment.
c) To comply with regulations.
d) To minimize the cost of waste disposal.

Answer: a) To reduce the risk of needlestick injuries. Explanation: The primary reason for safe handling and disposal of sharps is to reduce the risk of needlestick injuries, which can lead to transmission of bloodborne pathogens. Compliance with regulations and maintaining a clean environment are also important, but safety is the primary concern.

190. When dealing with a pediatric patient, what method might be effective in relieving their fear of needles?
a) Telling them it won't hurt.
b) Ignoring their fear.
c) Engaging them in a conversation or using distractions.
d) Rushing through the procedure.

Answer: c) Engaging them in a conversation or using distractions. Explanation: Talking to the child or using distractions like a toy or a story can help to alleviate their anxiety and make the procedure smoother for both the patient and the phlebotomist.

191. A patient with a history of fainting during blood draws is about to undergo phlebotomy. What is the best course of action?
a) Conduct the blood draw while the patient is in a seated position.
b) Have the patient stand up and walk around before the blood draw.
c) Have the patient in a lying position or ensure the chair has good support.
d) Advise the patient to hold their breath during the procedure.

Answer: c) Have the patient in a lying position or ensure the chair has good support.
Explanation: For patients with a history of fainting, it's advisable to conduct the blood draw in a lying position or a chair with good support to prevent injury in case they faint.

192. Which of the following factors can significantly affect the results of certain blood tests and should be considered during patient preparation?
a) Patient's zodiac sign.
b) Patient's favorite color.
c) Patient's diet and fasting state.
d) Patient's name.

Answer: c) Patient's diet and fasting state.
Explanation: A patient's diet and whether or not they have fasted can affect the results of certain blood tests, such as glucose and lipid panels.

193. What should be done if a patient refuses a blood draw?
a) Proceed anyway since it's for their health.
b) Bribe the patient.
c) Inform the patient of the importance, but respect their decision and inform the healthcare provider.
d) Threaten to call security.

Answer: c) Inform the patient of the importance, but respect their decision and inform the healthcare provider.
Explanation: It's important to respect patient autonomy. Inform them of the significance of the test, but if they refuse, it is important to respect their decision and notify the healthcare provider.

194. What is the best way to ensure correct patient identification before a blood draw?
a) Asking the patient's name.
b) Checking the patient's wristband.
c) Guessing based on appearance.
d) Asking a family member.

Answer: b) Checking the patient's wristband.
Explanation: Checking the patient's wristband and having the patient confirm their name and date of birth is the most reliable method for correct identification.

195. When preparing to draw blood from a patient who is cold, what measure might improve blood flow to the extremities?
a) Asking the patient to cross their arms.
b) Applying a warm compress.
c) Telling the patient to relax.
d) Rubbing hands together.

Answer: b) Applying a warm compress.
Explanation: Applying a warm compress can help to improve circulation and make the veins more accessible.

196. How can you prepare for a blood draw on a patient with difficult veins?
a) Use a larger needle to ensure success.
b) Have the patient do arm exercises.
c) Use a tourniquet and palpate for the best site, potentially using a smaller needle.
d) Guess and attempt multiple sites.

Answer: c) Use a tourniquet and palpate for the best site, potentially using a smaller needle.
Explanation: Using a tourniquet and taking the time to palpate for the most accessible vein, and considering the use of a smaller needle, can improve the chances of a successful blood draw with difficult veins.

197. Which of the following is an important aspect of patient preparation for a blood draw?
a) The patient must know the name of all phlebotomists in the lab.
b) The patient should be well-fed prior to the procedure.
c) The phlebotomist should ensure the patient understands the procedure.
d) The phlebotomist should give the patient an overview of their personal background.

Answer: c) The phlebotomist should ensure the patient understands the procedure.
Explanation: Clear communication with the patient, ensuring they understand the procedure and why it's being performed, is a crucial aspect of patient preparation.

198. In a case where a patient shows severe anxiety about the upcoming blood draw, what should the phlebotomist do?
a) Ignore the patient's anxiety and continue with the procedure.
b) Explain the importance of the test, try to calm the patient, and proceed when they feel ready.
c) Tell the patient that their fear is irrational.
d) Leave the patient alone to deal with their anxiety.

Answer: b) Explain the importance of the test, try to calm the patient, and proceed when they feel ready.
Explanation: It's crucial to address a patient's anxiety by explaining the importance of the test, attempting to soothe them, and only proceeding when they feel prepared.

199. What is the ideal site for an adult blood draw?
a) The antecubital area of the arm.
b) The tip of the index finger.
c) The heel of the foot.
d) The middle of the forearm.

Answer: a) The antecubital area of the arm.
Explanation: The antecubital area of the arm (inside of the elbow) is usually the best site for a blood draw because it typically has the largest and most accessible veins.

200. You are about to perform a venipuncture on an elderly patient with delicate, bruised skin. What's the best course of action?
a) Proceed as usual.
b) Use a larger needle to get it over with quickly.
c) Cancel the procedure.
d) Use a butterfly needle and be gentle to minimize trauma.

Answer: d) Use a butterfly needle and be gentle to minimize trauma.
Explanation: Elderly patients often have delicate skin. In such cases, using a smaller butterfly needle can help minimize trauma to the skin and underlying tissues. Gentle handling is also crucial to prevent bruising.

201. A child comes in for a blood draw and is visibly frightened. How should you handle this situation?
a) Ask the child to look away and proceed quickly.
b) Engage the child in conversation or use a distraction to ease their fear.
c) Ask the parent to hold the child down.
d) Cancel the procedure.

Answer: b) Engage the child in conversation or use a distraction to ease their fear.
Explanation: Children often fear needles. Distracting them with a conversation or a toy can help alleviate their anxiety, making the procedure easier for both the child and the phlebotomist.

202. A patient you've been asked to draw blood from is wearing a religious garment that covers the usual blood draw sites. How should you proceed?
a) Insist the patient removes the garment.
b) Cancel the blood draw.
c) Respectfully ask the patient if they can adjust their garment to access the site, explaining why.
d) Perform the blood draw through the garment.

Answer: c) Respectfully ask the patient if they can adjust their garment to access the site, explaining why.
Explanation: It's important to respect a patient's religious practices while also ensuring they receive the necessary medical care. A respectful conversation with the patient about why you need to access the area is the best approach.

203. Your patient is a professional pianist and asks you not to draw blood from his right arm. However, the veins in his left arm are not as visible. What is the best course of action?
a) Insist on drawing blood from the right arm.
b) Use a vein in the left arm, utilizing a warm compress if necessary.
c) Cancel the procedure.
d) Draw blood from his leg instead.

Answer: b) Use a vein in the left arm, utilizing a warm compress if necessary.
Explanation: As a healthcare professional, you should take into account the patient's occupation and lifestyle while causing minimum discomfort. Here, using a warm compress can improve blood flow, making the veins more accessible.

204. A diabetic patient comes for a fasting blood glucose test but admits they've had breakfast. What should you do?
a) Proceed with the test and note the incident.
b) Tell the patient to come back another day.
c) Perform the test but don't report the incident.
d) Tell the patient that eating breakfast doesn't affect the test.

Answer: a) Proceed with the test and note the incident.
Explanation: The test result could be influenced by the food the patient has consumed. It's necessary to perform the test as ordered by the physician, but it's crucial to note that the patient was not fasting so that the results can be interpreted correctly.

205. A patient has expressed anxiety about the impending blood draw. Which of the following actions should you take?
a) Proceed as usual.
b) Tell the patient to stop worrying.
c) Ask the patient to leave and come back when they are less anxious.
d) Take the time to explain the procedure, answer questions, and provide reassurances.

Answer: d) Take the time to explain the procedure, answer questions, and provide reassurances.
Explanation: Addressing a patient's anxiety is essential. Explaining the procedure, answering questions, and providing reassurance can help calm the patient and make the procedure easier.

206. You are about to draw blood from a patient but they appear pale and sweaty. What's the best course of action?
a) Proceed as usual.
b) Postpone the procedure and seek further advice.
c) Insist the patient is okay and continue.
d) Cancel the procedure.

Answer: b) Postpone the procedure and seek further advice.
Explanation: These could be signs of fear or a potential health problem, such as low blood sugar. It is best to postpone the procedure and seek advice to ensure patient safety.

207. A patient with no visible or palpable veins in the arms has come in for a routine blood draw. What should you do?
a) Try to find a vein in the legs.
b) Use the smallest needle and try to find a vein in the arms.
c) Rehydrate the patient and try again later.
d) Cancel the procedure.

Answer: c) Rehydrate the patient and try again later.
Explanation: Dehydration can make veins less visible or palpable. If no veins are apparent and the blood draw isn't urgent, rehydrating the patient and trying again later may help.

208. In preparing a patient for venipuncture, you notice a rash on the intended draw site. What is the best course of action?
a) Proceed with the blood draw.
b) Apply an ointment to the rash before proceeding.
c) Choose an alternative, healthy site for the venipuncture.
d) Cancel the procedure.

Answer: c) Choose an alternative, healthy site for the venipuncture.
Explanation: It's essential to avoid areas of the skin with rashes or other visible conditions, as these areas may be more susceptible to infection or could interfere with the venipuncture procedure. Always choose the healthiest possible site for blood draws.

209. When drawing blood from a patient, how should you confirm their identity?
a) By their room number.
b) By their appearance.
c) By asking them to confirm their name and date of birth.
d) By their assigned patient number.

Answer: c) By asking them to confirm their name and date of birth.

Explanation: A patient's identity should be confirmed by asking them to state their full name and date of birth. This is a more reliable method than relying on room numbers or appearance, which can change or be misleading.

210. In an outpatient setting, a patient provides you with their medical card for identification. What additional step should you take?
a) Take their word for it.
b) Ask them to verify their full name and date of birth.
c) Ask them for another form of identification.
d) Rely on the medical card only.

Answer: b) Ask them to verify their full name and date of birth.
Explanation: Even when presented with an identification card, it's important to have patients verbally confirm their identity by stating their full name and date of birth.

211. A patient who is unconscious is in need of an urgent blood draw. How can you confirm the patient's identity?
a) Rely on the patient's family to identify them.
b) Use the patient's ID bracelet.
c) Ask the nursing staff.
d) Check the patient's wallet.

Answer: b) Use the patient's ID bracelet.
Explanation: For unconscious patients, the patient's identification bracelet is the most reliable source of identification.

212. A patient's family member insists on confirming the patient's identity for them. How should you handle this situation?
a) Allow the family member to confirm the patient's identity.
b) Ask the patient to confirm their identity, if they are able to.
c) Use the patient's ID bracelet.
d) Ask the nursing staff.

Answer: b) Ask the patient to confirm their identity, if they are able to.
Explanation: If a patient is capable of speaking for themselves, it's important for them to confirm their own identity to avoid any potential confusion or mix-ups.

213. A patient tells you their nickname and insists on being identified by that name. How should you handle this situation?
a) Use the nickname for identification.
b) Ask the patient for their full, legal name.
c) Check the patient's ID bracelet.
d) Use the patient's assigned number.

Answer: b) Ask the patient for their full, legal name.
Explanation: For identification purposes, it's necessary to use the patient's full, legal name, regardless of any nicknames they may prefer.

214. What is one crucial step that should be taken to ensure patient identification during a phlebotomy procedure?
a) Memorizing the patient's face.
b) Checking the patient's ID bracelet and asking them to verify their full name and date of birth.
c) Matching the patient to the description in their medical records.
d) Relying on the patient's room number.

Answer: b) Checking the patient's ID bracelet and asking them to verify their full name and date of birth.
Explanation: The most reliable way to confirm a patient's identity is by checking their ID bracelet and having them verbally confirm their full name and date of birth. This helps avoid potential errors that can occur from relying on other methods of identification.

215. A patient has no ID bracelet and is unable to communicate. What should you do?
a) Proceed with the procedure based on their medical records.
b) Use facial recognition software.
c) Ask a family member or the nursing staff to confirm their identity.
d) Postpone the procedure until the patient's identity can be confirmed.

Answer: d) Postpone the procedure until the patient's identity can be confirmed.

216. You are about to draw blood from a patient in a hospital room. The patient's ID band is on the bedside table, not on their wrist. What is your next step?
a) Put the ID band on the patient and proceed.
b) Ask the patient to confirm their name and date of birth.
c) Proceed with the draw without confirming the patient's identity.
d) Ignore the ID band and ask the patient for their name.

Answer: b) Ask the patient to confirm their name and date of birth.
Explanation: The patient should always have the ID band on. However, in situations like this, asking the patient to verbally confirm their identity is the best approach to ensure accuracy.

217. A patient for a blood draw appears unconscious. How do you confirm their identity?
a) Proceed with the blood draw without confirmation.
b) Check the ID band and confirm with the nurse or caregiver.
c) Wake the patient up and ask for their name.
d) Cancel the blood draw.

Answer: b) Check the ID band and confirm with the nurse or caregiver.
Explanation: If a patient is unable to confirm their identity, you should use other reliable sources of information. The ID band is one such source, and confirming with a nurse or caregiver provides added assurance.

218. A non-English speaking patient comes in for a blood draw. How do you confirm their identity?
a) Ask them to write down their name and date of birth.
b) Use a translator or language line to confirm the patient's details.
c) Skip the identity confirmation and proceed with the blood draw.
d) Cancel the blood draw due to language barrier.

Answer: b) Use a translator or language line to confirm the patient's details.
Explanation: It's crucial to confirm a patient's identity, regardless of language barriers. Translators and language lines are valuable tools for ensuring clear communication in these situations.

219. Your patient for a blood draw is a newborn. What is the best way to confirm the baby's identity?
a) Check the baby's ID band and confirm with the mother or caregiver.
b) Ask the baby's name.
c) Proceed without confirmation.
d) Cancel the blood draw due to inability to confirm the identity.

Answer: a) Check the baby's ID band and confirm with the mother or caregiver.
Explanation: Newborns are identified using ID bands and confirmation from the mother or caregiver. These two methods together provide the most reliable confirmation of the baby's identity.

220. A child comes in for a blood draw accompanied by a woman who identifies herself as the child's nanny. How do you confirm the child's identity?
a) Ask the child for their name and date of birth.
b) Use the ID provided by the nanny.
c) Ask the nanny for the child's details.
d) Cancel the blood draw due to uncertainty of the identity.

Answer: a) Ask the child for their name and date of birth.
Explanation: The child (if able to speak and understand) can be a reliable source of their own identification information. However, it's also important to cross-reference with any ID or information provided by the nanny.

221. You are about to perform a blood draw on a patient but the name on the requisition form doesn't match the patient's verbal confirmation or the ID band. What should you do?
a) Proceed with the blood draw.
b) Confirm the patient's identity with a caregiver or family member.
c) Stop and resolve the discrepancy before proceeding.
d) Cancel the blood draw.

Answer: c) Stop and resolve the discrepancy before proceeding.
Explanation: It's important to resolve any discrepancies in a patient's identity before proceeding with the blood draw. This ensures the safety of the patient and the accuracy of the test results.

222. You are performing a blood draw at a nursing home. The patient is asleep, and their ID band is partially obscured. What is the best next step?
a) Awaken the patient and ask for their name.
b) Consult the nursing home staff for identification.
c) Proceed with the blood draw as you assume this is the correct patient.
d) Check the room number and match it with the information on the requisition form.

Answer: b) Consult the nursing home staff for identification.
Explanation: In this case, it would be ideal to confirm the patient's identity through the nursing home staff who are familiar with the patient. This will ensure you are performing the procedure on the correct individual.

223. A phlebotomist is preparing to collect a blood sample from a patient whose ID band is missing. How should they proceed?
a) Ask the patient to confirm their identity by stating their name and birth date.
b) Proceed with the blood draw, assuming that the patient's identity matches the requisition form.
c) Ask a nurse or healthcare provider to verify the patient's identity.
d) Discontinue the process until an ID band can be provided.

Answer: d) Discontinue the process until an ID band can be provided.
Explanation: If the ID band is missing, the phlebotomist should stop and ensure that a new band is provided. It's critical to the safety and accuracy of the procedure that the patient's identity is confirmed.

224. The phlebotomist has two patients with the same first and last name. How should they proceed with identifying each patient correctly?
a) Confirm the patient's name and birth date.
b) Ask the nurse to identify the patients.
c) Check the middle name or initial.
d) All of the above.

Answer: d) All of the above.
Explanation: Multiple points of data should be used to distinguish patients with the same name. These could include middle names, birth dates, and nurse confirmation.

225. During a busy morning at the clinic, a phlebotomist notices that the patient's ID band information partially matches the requisition form. What should be the next step?
a) Proceed with the blood draw as they have similar information.
b) Ask the patient to confirm their identity by stating their name and birth date.
c) Confirm with the nurse or healthcare provider.
d) Use the patient's verbal confirmation to proceed with the blood draw.

Answer: c) Confirm with the nurse or healthcare provider.
Explanation: If there's any discrepancy between the ID band and the requisition form, it's crucial to validate the information with another healthcare professional before proceeding.

226. A pediatric patient's mother insists that you don't need to check the child's ID band as she can confirm her child's identity. What should you do?
a) Trust the mother's confirmation and proceed with the blood draw.
b) Check the child's ID band anyway.
c) Ask the nurse to confirm the child's identity.
d) Cancel the blood draw as the patient's identity can't be confirmed.

Answer: b) Check the child's ID band anyway.
Explanation: Regardless of a parent or caregiver's assurance, it's essential to follow proper patient identification procedures. This involves checking the child's ID band.

227. When collecting a blood sample from an unconscious patient, what should a phlebotomist do to ensure correct identification?
a) Ask a family member for the patient's information.
b) Use the information provided on the requisition form.
c) Check the patient's ID band.
d) Guess the patient's identity based on their appearance.

Answer: c) Check the patient's ID band.
Explanation: The ID band is the most reliable source of patient information in such a situation, especially when the patient is unable to verbally confirm their identity.

228. During a routine blood draw, you encounter a patient with no identification band. What should you do?
a) Ask the patient for their name and date of birth.
b) Proceed with the blood draw.
c) Ask a nurse to identify the patient.
d) Wait until an identification band is placed on the patient.

Answer: d) Wait until an identification band is placed on the patient.
Explanation: Proper patient identification is crucial to healthcare safety. The patient's identity should be confirmed using an ID band before proceeding with any procedure.

229. You are about to perform a blood draw and the patient's name on the ID band is slightly different from the name on the lab requisition. What should you do?
a) Assume they are the same person and proceed.
b) Ask the patient to confirm their name.
c) Check with the patient's nurse for clarification.
d) Wait until the discrepancy is resolved before proceeding.

Answer: d) Wait until the discrepancy is resolved before proceeding.
Explanation: Any discrepancy in the patient's identity must be resolved before proceeding with the procedure to ensure the correct patient is being treated.

230. What is an appropriate way to verify a patient's identity if they cannot communicate verbally and do not have an ID band?
a) Proceed with the blood draw and confirm the identity later.
b) Ask a family member or caregiver.
c) Use facial recognition.
d) Do not proceed with the blood draw.

Answer: b) Ask a family member or caregiver.
Explanation: When a patient can't communicate verbally, other reliable sources such as family members or caregivers can provide necessary confirmation of identity.

231. A patient with Alzheimer's disease cannot confirm their identity. How should you proceed?
a) Ask the patient repeatedly until they remember.
b) Use the ID band and confirm with a nurse or caregiver.
c) Cancel the blood draw due to the patient's inability to confirm their identity.
d) Assume the patient's identity based on room number.

Answer: b) Use the ID band and confirm with a nurse or caregiver.
Explanation: For patients who cannot communicate effectively, the ID band is a crucial tool for confirming identity. Cross-checking with a nurse or caregiver provides added assurance.

232. What should you do if a patient's ID band falls off during a blood draw?
a) Continue with the blood draw, as you have already confirmed the patient's identity.
b) Stop and replace the ID band before continuing.
c) Ask the patient to hold their ID band.
d) Continue the blood draw and replace the ID band afterward.

Answer: b) Stop and replace the ID band before continuing.
Explanation: An ID band is a crucial element of patient safety. If it falls off, it should be replaced before continuing with any procedure.

233. You are drawing blood from an infant. How can you verify the infant's identity?
a) Ask the parent to confirm the infant's name and birth date.
b) Check the crib card and the infant's ID band.
c) Ask the nurse.
d) All of the above.

Answer: d) All of the above.
Explanation: In the case of infants, multiple sources of confirmation, including the parent, crib card, ID band, and nurse can be used to confirm identity.

234. What is the minimum amount of identifying information you should confirm before proceeding with a blood draw?
a) First and last name.
b) First name and date of birth.
c) Last name and date of birth.
d) First and last name and date of birth.

Answer: d) First and last name and date of birth.
Explanation: The most reliable way to confirm a patient's identity is to verify at least two pieces of identifying information, typically the patient's full name and date of birth.

235. During a blood draw, the patient informs you that they have a nickname listed on their ID band. What should you do?
a) Use the nickname for identification.
b) Ask the patient to confirm their legal name and date of birth.
c) Ignore the nickname and use the name listed on the ID band.
d) Confirm the nickname with a nurse or caregiver.

Answer: b) Ask the patient to confirm their legal name and date of birth.
Explanation: Always use the legal name and date of birth for patient identification, even if the patient prefers to be called by a nickname.

236. You are asked to draw blood from a patient who is sedated and unable to confirm their identity. What is your best course of action?
a) Proceed with the blood draw using the name on the requisition form.
b) Ask the patient's family member or caregiver to confirm the patient's identity.
c) Check the patient's ID band and confirm with the nurse.
d) Cancel the blood draw.

Answer: c) Check the patient's ID band and confirm with the nurse.
Explanation: The ID band is a reliable source of patient information, and the nurse can provide additional confirmation.

237. You have two patients in the same room with similar names. How do you correctly identify the patient for a blood draw?
a) Ask the patients to confirm their names.
b) Compare the names on the requisition form with the names on the ID bands.
c) Ask the nurse to identify the correct patient.
d) All of the above.

Answer: d) All of the above.
Explanation: With similar patient names, multiple methods of identification should be used to avoid mix-ups. This includes the requisition form, ID bands, and a nurse's confirmation.

238. During a blood draw, you accidentally use an expired tube. What is the potential error and consequence?
a) The tube may not draw blood correctly, resulting in a faulty sample.
b) The results will automatically be incorrect.
c) The tube will be dangerous to the patient.
d) There will be no consequence as long as the blood is drawn properly.

Answer: a) The tube may not draw blood correctly, resulting in a faulty sample.
Explanation: An expired tube can affect the quality of the sample, potentially leading to inaccurate results.

239. What can happen if a tourniquet is left on a patient's arm for too long during a blood draw?
a) There will be no effect on the patient.
b) It may result in hemoconcentration.
c) The patient will experience extreme pain.
d) It will improve the quality of the sample.

Answer: b) It may result in hemoconcentration.
Explanation: Leaving a tourniquet on for too long can cause hemoconcentration, a potential error that can distort laboratory results.

240. What could be the consequence of mislabeling a blood sample?
a) The sample could be identified as belonging to another patient.
b) The lab will automatically reject the sample.
c) The patient will have to have their blood drawn again.
d) All of the above.

Answer: d) All of the above.
Explanation: Mislabeling a blood sample can lead to multiple consequences, including patient misidentification, sample rejection, and the need for re-drawing the sample.

241. In the case of needlestick injury, what is the potential error and consequence?
a) No potential error or consequence.
b) Potential infection to the healthcare provider.
c) Risk of fainting.
d) The patient may feel pain.

Answer: b) Potential infection to the healthcare provider.
Explanation: Needlestick injuries pose a significant risk of infection, especially from bloodborne pathogens, to the healthcare provider.

242. What can be the potential error and consequence of not obtaining informed consent before a blood draw?
a) There will be no error or consequence.
b) The patient may feel uncomfortable.
c) Legal and ethical consequences.
d) Poor quality of the sample.

Answer: c) Legal and ethical consequences.
Explanation: Not obtaining informed consent can result in legal and ethical issues, as it is a patient's right to understand and consent to any procedure.

243. If the order of draw is not correctly followed, what could be the potential error and consequence?
a) Incorrect test results.
b) Patient discomfort.
c) Needlestick injury.
d) No potential error or consequence.

Answer: a) Incorrect test results.
Explanation: Not following the correct order of draw can lead to cross-contamination of additives between tubes, potentially affecting test results.

244. In a situation where you are dealing with an elderly patient with fragile veins, what is the most suitable needle gauge to use?
a) 16 gauge
b) 18 gauge
c) 21 gauge
d) 23 gauge

Answer: d) 23 gauge
Explanation: For elderly patients with fragile veins, a smaller needle gauge (higher number) such as 23 is often more suitable to prevent vein damage.

245. Which type of blood collection device would be most appropriate for a difficult venipuncture where the veins are not easily palpable?
a) Evacuated tube system
b) Winged infusion set
c) Syringe system
d) Capillary tubes

Answer: b) Winged infusion set
Explanation: Winged infusion sets, also known as "butterfly needles", provide better control and are often used for difficult venipunctures, such as in patients with small or fragile veins.

246. What type of equipment would be best suited for the collection of a large volume of blood?
a) Capillary tube
b) Syringe
c) Microtube
d) Vacutainer tube

Answer: d) Vacutainer tube
Explanation: Vacutainer tubes are capable of holding larger volumes of blood, which is suitable when a large volume is required for testing.

247. Which of the following tubes would be best for glucose testing?
a) Red top tube
b) Blue top tube
c) Grey top tube
d) Green top tube

Answer: c) Grey top tube
Explanation: Grey top tubes contain sodium fluoride, which inhibits glycolysis, and are used for glucose testing to provide accurate readings.

248. For a patient with a known clotting disorder, which blood collection tube would be the most suitable?
a) Red top tube
b) Light blue top tube
c) Green top tube
d) Lavender top tube

Answer: b) Light blue top tube
Explanation: Light blue top tubes contain sodium citrate, an anticoagulant that helps to prevent clotting, making it a suitable choice for patients with clotting disorders.

249. Which equipment is most appropriate for a capillary puncture on a newborn?
a) Standard needle and syringe
b) Evacuated tube system
c) Capillary tube and lancet
d) Butterfly needle

Answer: c) Capillary tube and lancet
Explanation: For newborns, a capillary puncture is often the preferred method, and this requires a capillary tube and lancet.

250. When would a phlebotomist select to use a needle with a smaller gauge number?
a) When veins are difficult to locate.
b) When a larger amount of blood is needed quickly.
c) When a patient has a fear of needles.
d) When a patient's veins are fragile.

Answer: b) When a larger amount of blood is needed quickly.
Explanation: The smaller the gauge number, the larger the needle. A larger needle allows for a faster blood draw when a large amount is needed quickly.

251. Which blood collection tube should be used for a complete blood count (CBC)?
a) Red top tube
b) Blue top tube
c) Lavender top tube
d) Green top tube

Answer: c) Lavender top tube
Explanation: The lavender top tube contains an anticoagulant that mixes with the blood to prevent it from clotting, preserving the cellular components necessary for a CBC.

252. In a situation where a patient has small or fragile veins, what equipment would be most appropriate?
a) Standard-sized needle
b) Winged infusion set
c) Vacutainer holder
d) Tourniquet
Answer: b) Winged infusion set

Explanation: A winged infusion set, also known as a butterfly needle, is often used for patients with small or fragile veins because it allows for more delicate control during the venipuncture procedure.

253. When would a phlebotomist most likely use a lancet?
a) To collect blood from an artery
b) To collect blood from an infant's heel
c) To collect blood from a vein
d) To collect blood from a finger

Answer: b) To collect blood from an infant's heel. Explanation: A lancet is a small device equipped with a needle used to make punctures, such as for blood sampling or for testing glucose levels. It is commonly used for heel sticks on infants.

254. What is the main purpose of a tourniquet in the phlebotomy procedure?
a) To stop bleeding after the procedure
b) To help find a suitable vein for venipuncture
c) To sterilize the skin before the procedure
d) To hold the collection tube

Answer: b) To help find a suitable vein for venipuncture Explanation: A tourniquet is applied around the upper arm to exert pressure and temporarily slow the flow of blood. This makes veins below the tourniquet larger and easier to locate.

255. If a phlebotomist plans to draw blood from a patient with a good, accessible vein, what would be the best choice of equipment?
a) Lancet
b) Winged infusion set
c) Vacuum tube
d) Evacuated collection tube system

Answer: d) Evacuated collection tube system Explanation: An evacuated collection tube system, which includes a holder and double-pointed needle, is a common choice for venipuncture in adults with good veins.

256. A phlebotomist plans to perform a blood draw on a patient with a high risk of fainting. What piece of equipment might be useful in this situation?
a) An extra-large needle
b) A butterfly needle
c) A phlebotomy chair
d) A tourniquet

Answer: c) A phlebotomy chair Explanation: A phlebotomy chair, particularly one that can be reclined, can be beneficial for patients who are prone to fainting during blood draws.

257. For a difficult venipuncture procedure, what piece of equipment can assist in visualizing veins?
a) A vein viewer
b) A tourniquet
c) A butterfly needle
d) A sharps container

Answer: a) A vein viewer Explanation: A vein viewer uses infrared technology to visualize veins, making it easier to find a suitable vein in difficult cases.

258. When should a phlebotomist use an alcohol swab?
a) Before applying the tourniquet
b) After removing the needle
c) To clean the site before venipuncture
d) To clean the needle before venipuncture

Answer: c) To clean the site before venipuncture Explanation: An alcohol swab is used to clean the venipuncture site before the procedure to prevent infection.

259. When a phlebotomist is selecting a vein for venipuncture, what is the most important criteria to consider?
a) The vein is close to the surface of the skin.
b) The vein is at least 1 inch away from an artery.
c) The vein is visible to the naked eye.
d) The vein is large enough to safely puncture with a needle.

Answer: d) The vein is large enough to safely puncture with a needle. Explanation: While it's beneficial if a vein is near the skin surface and visible, the most important factor is that it's large enough to safely puncture with a needle, minimizing discomfort and the risk of complications for the patient.

260. A phlebotomist is performing venipuncture on a patient with dehydration. What should the phlebotomist be especially careful to avoid?
a) Selecting a vein that is too small.
b) Selecting a vein that is too large.
c) Selecting a vein that is too close to the surface of the skin.
d) Selecting a vein that is visible to the naked eye.

Answer: a) Selecting a vein that is too small. Explanation: Dehydration may cause veins to become smaller and more difficult to puncture. Selecting a vein that is too small may lead to a failed attempt at blood collection or harm to the patient.

261. When performing venipuncture, what should a phlebotomist do if a vein is difficult to locate?
a) Use a larger needle.
b) Apply a warm compress to the area.
c) Use a vein in the patient's foot.
d) Attempt to puncture the skin where they believe a vein should be.

Answer: b) Apply a warm compress to the area. Explanation: Applying a warm compress can help dilate the veins and make them easier to locate.

262. What is the best practice when choosing between two veins that are equal in size and accessibility?
a) Choose the vein that is further from the heart.
b) Choose the vein on the dominant side of the patient's body.
c) Choose the vein on the non-dominant side of the patient's body.
d) The choice between the two veins doesn't matter.

Answer: c) Choose the vein on the non-dominant side of the patient's body. Explanation: The non-dominant side is generally used for venipuncture to avoid causing discomfort in the patient's dominant arm.

263. When selecting a vein for venipuncture, why should a phlebotomist avoid an area where the vein crosses over a joint?
a) The needle may accidentally puncture the joint.
b) It can cause increased pain for the patient.
c) The joint may cause the vein to move during the procedure.
d) All of the above.

Answer: d) All of the above. Explanation: Areas where veins cross over joints should be avoided because the movement of the joint can cause the vein to move, increasing the risk of an unsuccessful puncture or causing discomfort for the patient. There's also a risk of accidentally puncturing the joint.

264. In preparing a patient for a phlebotomy procedure, the phlebotomist should:
a) Explain the procedure in technical medical jargon to show expertise.
b) Minimize communication to reduce the patient's anxiety.
c) Explain the procedure in layman's terms and answer any questions the patient may have.
d) Proceed with the procedure without explanation as it is routine.

Answer: c) Explain the procedure in layman's terms and answer any questions the patient may have. Explanation: Clear, simple communication helps alleviate patient anxiety and ensures informed consent.

265. When a patient expresses fear about the upcoming venipuncture, how should a phlebotomist respond?
a) Tell the patient not to worry and proceed with the procedure.
b) Sympathize with the patient and validate their feelings before proceeding.
c) Ignore the patient's fear to avoid escalating the situation.
d) Tell the patient that they are overreacting.

Answer: b) Sympathize with the patient and validate their feelings before proceeding. Explanation: Validating the patient's feelings and showing empathy can help alleviate their fears and build a sense of trust.

266. A patient is reluctant to undergo a venipuncture procedure. What should the phlebotomist do?
a) Insist that the procedure is important and must be done.
b) Explain the necessity of the test and address any concerns the patient might have.
c) Proceed with the procedure without the patient's consent.
d) Inform the patient's doctor and leave the room.

Answer: b) Explain the necessity of the test and address any concerns the patient might have.
Explanation: A phlebotomist should ensure the patient understands the procedure and its necessity while addressing their concerns.

267. If a patient asks about their test results, the phlebotomist should:
a) Provide a detailed explanation of what they believe the results mean.
b) Refer the patient to their healthcare provider for a discussion of the results.
c) Tell the patient that they are not allowed to view their results.
d) Avoid answering the question.

Answer: b) Refer the patient to their healthcare provider for a discussion of the results. Explanation: While phlebotomists play a critical role in sample collection, interpretation of test results falls under the provider's scope.

268. Prior to performing a venipuncture, what is an important step in preparing the patient?
a) Having the patient lift weights to increase vein visibility.
b) Informing the patient to look directly at the needle during insertion.
c) Asking the patient to make a fist to facilitate vein location.
d) Ignoring the patient's anxiety as it's a common reaction.

Answer: c) Asking the patient to make a fist to facilitate vein location. Explanation: Having the patient make a fist (without "pumping" the hand, which can affect test results) can help the phlebotomist locate suitable veins for venipuncture.

269. When working with a pediatric patient, the phlebotomist should:
a) Speak primarily with the child, ignoring the parent.
b) Speak primarily with the parent, ignoring the child.
c) Address both the child and the parent, explaining the procedure at an appropriate level for each.
d) Proceed with the procedure without explanation to avoid frightening the child.

Answer: c) Address both the child and the parent, explaining the procedure at an appropriate level for each. Explanation: It's important to communicate effectively with both the child and the parent. This helps ease anxiety and ensure understanding of the procedure.

270. A phlebotomist needs to draw blood from a non-English speaking patient. What is the best course of action?
a) Use hand gestures to communicate.
b) Speak slowly and loudly in English.
c) Get a family member to interpret.
d) Use an authorized medical interpreter or language line.

Answer: d) Use an authorized medical interpreter or language line. Explanation: Professional medical interpreters are trained to accurately communicate complex medical information. Relying on family members or attempting to communicate through hand gestures can lead to misunderstandings.

271. If a patient faints during a blood draw, the phlebotomist should:
a) Stop the draw, lower the patient's head, and seek immediate assistance.
b) Continue with the draw since the patient is already unconscious.
c) Leave the room to find a nurse or doctor.
d) Lay the patient flat without seeking assistance.

Answer: a) Stop the draw, lower the patient's head, and seek immediate assistance. Explanation: Patient safety is paramount. If a patient faints, stop the procedure, ensure the patient is in a safe position, and get help.

272. In preparing a geriatric patient for a blood draw, a phlebotomist should:
a) Talk loudly assuming the patient has hearing problems.
b) Limit communication assuming the patient has cognitive impairments.
c) Use a one-size-fits-all approach since all geriatric patients are similar.
d) Treat the patient with patience and respect, acknowledging potential age-related physical or cognitive limitations.

Answer: d) Treat the patient with patience and respect, acknowledging potential age-related physical or cognitive limitations. Explanation: Geriatric patients often have unique needs that require patience, respect, and an individualized approach.

273. If a patient refuses a blood draw, the phlebotomist should:
a) Proceed with the draw, stating that it's doctor's orders.
b) Leave the room immediately without saying anything.
c) Force the patient to comply for their own good.
d) Respect the patient's wishes, inform the provider, and document the refusal.

Answer: d) Respect the patient's wishes, inform the provider, and document the refusal. Explanation: A patient has the right to refuse treatment. The phlebotomist should respect this, inform the appropriate healthcare provider, and ensure the refusal is properly documented.

274. When drawing blood from a pediatric patient who is crying and agitated, a useful strategy might be to:
a) Ignore the crying and proceed as usual.
b) Use a distraction toy or device.
c) Tell the child to stop crying because it won't hurt.
d) Threaten the child with a longer procedure if they don't stop crying.

Answer: b) Use a distraction toy or device. Explanation: Distraction can be a very effective technique to help ease a child's fear and anxiety during a procedure.

275. What is the best way to position an anxious patient to make them feel more comfortable during a blood draw?
a) Have them stand to assert dominance.
b) Have them lie down and close their eyes.
c) Allow them to sit in a comfortable, secure chair.
d) Position does not matter as long as the procedure is done quickly.

Answer: c) Allow them to sit in a comfortable, secure chair. Explanation: A comfortable, secure sitting position can help an anxious patient feel safer and more at ease.

276. A patient starts to feel dizzy during a blood draw. As a phlebotomist, you should:
a) Continue the draw quickly to finish as soon as possible.
b) Immediately stop the draw, ensure the patient is safe, and apply a cold compress to the forehead.
c) Ignore the patient's complaints and proceed.
d) Ask the patient to shake it off and remain still.

Answer: b) Immediately stop the draw, ensure the patient is safe, and apply a cold compress to the forehead. Explanation: Patient's safety and comfort is a priority. When a patient feels unwell during a procedure, the phlebotomist should stop and provide care.

277. A technique that can be used to minimize discomfort for patients when performing a venipuncture is to:
a) Insert the needle as quickly as possible.
b) Use a larger needle to make sure the procedure is done quickly.
c) Insert the needle at an angle larger than 30 degrees.
d) Apply a local anesthetic cream, if approved and available.

Answer: d) Apply a local anesthetic cream, if approved and available. Explanation: Local anesthetic creams can be used to numb the skin and decrease pain during needle procedures.

278. For a patient with a fear of needles, which strategy might be most helpful to ease their anxiety?
a) Tell them to look away during the procedure.
b) Tell them their fear is irrational.
c) Quickly perform the procedure without warning.
d) Insist they watch to overcome their fear.

Answer: a) Tell them to look away during the procedure. Explanation: For patients with a fear of needles, it can be helpful to suggest they look away during the procedure.

279. Which method can effectively distract a patient during a blood draw?
a) Discussing the details of the procedure.
b) Having a casual conversation or asking about their day.
c) Discussing other patients' reactions to blood draws.
d) Discussing the risks associated with blood draws.

Answer: b) Having a casual conversation or asking about their day. Explanation: Engaging the patient in light conversation can serve as a distraction and make the patient feel more at ease.

280. If a patient has a history of fainting during blood draws, a useful approach may be to:
a) Tell them fainting is uncommon and they shouldn't worry.
b) Have them lay down during the procedure.
c) Ask them to stand up to get it over with quickly.
d) Tell them their fear is irrational and they should control it.

Answer: b) Have them lay down during the procedure. Explanation: Lying down can help prevent fainting by improving blood flow to the brain, making it a good option for patients who have a history of fainting.

281. A patient is nervous about the pain of a blood draw. Which of the following can help ease their concern?
a) Assure them that the pain is insignificant and they're overreacting.
b) Show them the size of the needle to prove it's not big.
c) Use a smaller gauge needle, if suitable and available.
d) Hurry to finish the procedure quickly, disregarding their feelings.

Answer: c) Use a smaller gauge needle, if suitable and available. Explanation: Using a smaller gauge needle can help reduce the pain of the puncture, easing patient's concern.

282. What can help a patient with a fear of blood to cope during a blood draw?
a) Have them watch the procedure to face their fear.
b) Advise them to close their eyes and take slow, deep breaths.
c) Show them the blood in the tube to prove it's not a lot.
d) Discuss the color and consistency of blood to distract them.

Answer: b) Advise them to close their eyes and take slow, deep breaths. Explanation: For a patient with a fear of blood, it can be helpful to suggest they close their eyes and use calming breathing techniques during the procedure.

283. When dealing with an anxious child, what strategy might help to create a more positive experience?
a) Conduct the procedure as quickly as possible, ignoring their feelings.
b) Provide a reward, such as a sticker or a small toy, after the procedure.
c) Ask the child to stop crying and be brave.
d) Threaten with a punishment if they don't cooperate.

Answer: b) Provide a reward, such as a sticker or a small toy, after the procedure. Explanation: A small reward after the procedure can turn a potentially negative experience into a more positive one, helping to ease fear and anxiety in children.

284. When selecting a venipuncture site, the first choice is typically the:
a) Femoral vein
b) Jugular vein
c) Median cubital vein
d) Dorsal metacarpal veins

Answer: c) Median cubital vein. Explanation: The median cubital vein in the antecubital fossa is typically the first choice for venipuncture due to its size, location, and relative ease of access.

285. What should be the primary concern when selecting a venipuncture site?
a) Convenience for the phlebotomist
b) Speed of blood flow
c) Patient comfort and safety
d) Visibility of the vein

Answer: c) Patient comfort and safety. Explanation: While all factors can play a part, the primary concern should always be the comfort and safety of the patient.

286. If a patient has a previously used site with visible bruises, it is recommended to:
a) Use the same site to avoid creating another puncture
b) Choose a site as far away as possible
c) Avoid the site and select a different, suitable location
d) Choose the same arm but a different site

Answer: c) Avoid the site and select a different, suitable location. Explanation: A bruised site indicates tissue damage, and repeated punctures could cause further harm.

287. If the median cubital vein is not accessible, which of the following veins should be considered next?
a) Basilic vein
b) Brachial vein
c) Cephalic vein
d) Radial vein

Answer: c) Cephalic vein. Explanation: If the median cubital vein is not accessible, the cephalic vein is often considered the next best option due to its size and location.

288. The first step in preparing a venipuncture site is to:
a) Palpate the vein
b) Apply the tourniquet
c) Cleanse the area with an antiseptic
d) Open the needle package

Answer: b) Apply the tourniquet. Explanation: Applying the tourniquet is the first step as it helps veins become more visible and palpable.

289. What is an important step after cleansing the venipuncture site but before needle insertion?
a) Checking patient's ID again
b) Allowing the antiseptic to dry
c) Removing the tourniquet
d) Asking the patient about their day

Answer: b) Allowing the antiseptic to dry. Explanation: Allowing the antiseptic to dry prevents stinging sensation for the patient and also ensures maximum effectiveness of the antiseptic.

290. Which veins should be avoided in the elderly due to the risk of thrombosis?
a) Median cubital veins
b) Cephalic veins
c) Basilic veins
d) Dorsal metacarpal veins

Answer: c) Basilic veins. Explanation: Basilic veins are deep and more susceptible to thrombosis; they should be avoided, especially in elderly patients.

291. In a patient with a bilateral mastectomy, which site would be appropriate for a venipuncture?
a) Basilic vein of either arm
b) Median cubital vein of either arm
c) Dorsal metacarpal veins of either hand
d) None of the above

Answer: c) Dorsal metacarpal veins of either hand. Explanation: After a bilateral mastectomy, blood should not be drawn from either arm. The dorsal metacarpal veins in the hands are the next best option.

292. If a patient has a strong pulse in the antecubital fossa, which action is most appropriate?
a) Proceed with the venipuncture, the pulse will not affect the collection
b) Use a smaller needle to avoid the artery
c) Select a different site, as a pulse may indicate an artery
d) Use a butterfly needle to give better control

Answer: c) Select a different site, as a pulse may indicate an artery. Explanation: A strong pulse in the area could indicate the presence of an artery rather than a vein. Accidental arterial puncture should be avoided.

293. When should you release the tourniquet during a venipuncture procedure?
a) Before the needle is inserted
b) Immediately after the needle is inserted
c) After the first tube of blood begins to fill
d) Within 1-2 minutes after it has been applied

Answer: d) Within 1-2 minutes after it has been applied. Explanation: The tourniquet should be released within 1-2 minutes after application to avoid hemoconcentration and potential changes in test results.

294. During venipuncture, the first tube drawn is typically for which type of tests?
a) Coagulation studies
b) Blood cultures
c) Chemistry tests
d) Hematology tests

Answer: b) Blood cultures. Explanation: Blood cultures are typically drawn first to avoid contamination from the needle or other substances that could affect the test results.

295. Which vein is most commonly used for venipuncture?
a) Median cubital vein
b) Basilic vein
c) Cephalic vein
d) Brachial vein

Answer: a) Median cubital vein. Explanation: The median cubital vein, located in the middle of the forearm, is usually the first choice for venipuncture due to its size and easy accessibility.

296. Which of the following veins are located in the antecubital fossa of the arm?
a) Median cubital, basilic, and cephalic veins
b) Jugular, subclavian, and axillary veins
c) Femoral, popliteal, and saphenous veins
d) Radial, ulnar, and interosseous veins

Answer: a) Median cubital, basilic, and cephalic veins. Explanation: The antecubital fossa of the arm houses the median cubital, basilic, and cephalic veins. These veins are commonly used for phlebotomy procedures.

297. What is the recommended maximum depth for a heel stick on a newborn?
a) 0.65 mm
b) 1.65 mm
c) 2.00 mm
d) 2.4 mm

Answer: c) 2.00 mm. Explanation: The recommended maximum depth for a heel stick on a newborn is 2.0 mm to prevent injury to the bone.

298. In the order of draw, which tube is typically drawn immediately after the tube for coagulation studies?
a) EDTA tube
b) Sodium citrate tube
c) Heparin tube
d) SST tube

Answer: d) SST tube. Explanation: Following the coagulation tube, which is typically a light-blue top sodium citrate tube, the SST (Serum Separator Tube) or "tiger top" tube is usually drawn next in the order of draw.

299. The smallest veins in the human body are known as:
a) Arterioles
b) Capillaries
c) Venules
d) Sinusoids

Answer: c) Venules. Explanation: Venules are the smallest veins in the body. They receive blood from the capillaries and drain into the larger veins.

300. In an adult patient, the correct angle for needle insertion during a venipuncture is:
a) 15 to 30 degrees
b) 30 to 45 degrees
c) 45 to 60 degrees
d) 60 to 75 degrees

Answer: a) 15 to 30 degrees. Explanation: The correct angle for needle insertion during a venipuncture in an adult is between 15 to 30 degrees.

301. The clear, yellowish fluid that remains after a blood clot forms is called:
a) Plasma
b) Serum
c) Hemolymph
d) Lymph

Answer: b) Serum. Explanation: Serum is the clear, yellowish fluid that remains after a blood clot forms. It is similar to plasma but lacks clotting factors.

302. Which white blood cells are primarily responsible for producing antibodies?
a) Neutrophils
b) Eosinophils
c) Lymphocytes
d) Monocytes

Answer: c) Lymphocytes. Explanation: Lymphocytes are primarily responsible for immune responses, including the production of antibodies.

303. When a tourniquet is applied to a patient's arm for a venipuncture, it should be:
a) Above the elbow
b) Below the elbow
c) Above the wrist
d) On the forearm

Answer: a) Above the elbow. Explanation: The tourniquet is typically placed above the elbow to help dilate the veins in the antecubital fossa, making them more visible and accessible for venipuncture.

304. Why are veins generally preferred over arteries for venipuncture?
a) Arteries have more nerve endings than veins
b) Veins are located closer to the skin surface
c) Blood flow in veins is slower than in arteries
d) All of the above

Answer: d) All of the above. Explanation: Veins are typically selected for venipuncture because they have fewer nerve endings (resulting in less pain), they are closer to the surface of the skin, and the blood flow in veins is slower than in arteries.

305. Which of the following veins is not usually suitable for venipuncture?
a) Median cubital vein
b) Femoral vein
c) Basilic vein
d) Cephalic vein

Answer: b) Femoral vein. Explanation: The femoral vein, located in the groin area, is not typically used for venipuncture due to its deep location and close proximity to the femoral artery and nerve.

306. What is the primary reason to avoid using the basilic vein as the first choice for venipuncture?
a) It is more sensitive to needle insertion
b) It is often more difficult to locate
c) It is in close proximity to the brachial artery and median nerve
d) It has a smaller diameter compared to other veins

Answer: c) It is in close proximity to the brachial artery and median nerve. Explanation: Although the basilic vein can be used for venipuncture, it is not usually the first choice due to its location near the brachial artery and median nerve, increasing the risk of injury.

307. What is the significance of the antecubital area in venipuncture?
a) It contains the largest vein in the body
b) It is the least painful area for venipuncture
c) It houses veins that are near the surface and well anchored
d) It offers the fastest blood flow for venipuncture

Answer: c) It houses veins that are near the surface and well anchored. Explanation: The antecubital area, located at the inside of the elbow, is often chosen for venipuncture because it contains veins that are near the surface, well anchored, and usually large enough for successful venipuncture.

308. Which layer of the blood vessel is composed primarily of smooth muscle and elastic fibers?
a) Tunica intima
b) Tunica media
c) Tunica adventitia
d) Tunica externa

Answer: b) Tunica media. Explanation: The tunica media, the middle layer of a blood vessel, is primarily composed of smooth muscle and elastic fibers. It helps control the diameter and blood flow of the vessel.

309. Why is it important to understand the valve locations in the veins when performing venipuncture?
a) To avoid puncturing a valve which can cause patient discomfort and yield a poor blood sample
b) Valves indicate the start of a new vein segment
c) Valves are more resilient to needle punctures
d) Valves can aid in blood collection by promoting blood flow into the collection tube

Answer: a) To avoid puncturing a valve which can cause patient discomfort and yield a poor blood sample. Explanation: Understanding valve locations can help the phlebotomist avoid these structures during venipuncture. Puncturing a valve can cause patient discomfort and potentially result in an insufficient blood sample.

310. During venipuncture, what role does the tourniquet play?
a) It decreases blood flow to the heart
b) It causes vasodilation in the forearm
c) It increases venous filling
d) All of the above

Answer: c) It increases venous filling. Explanation: The tourniquet is applied to increase venous filling by impeding venous flow. This makes the veins below the tourniquet more prominent and easier to puncture.

311. What is the role of the erythrocytes (red blood cells) in the blood?
a) They help in clotting
b) They carry oxygen from the lungs to the body's cells
c) They fight infections
d) They regulate blood pH

Answer: b) They carry oxygen from the lungs to the body's cells. Explanation: Erythrocytes, or red blood cells, primarily function to transport oxygen from the lungs to the body's tissues.

312. When collecting blood samples for glucose testing, why is the patient typically asked to fast?
a) Because food can alter the pH of the blood
b) Because eating triggers the release of hormones that can affect glucose levels
c) Because food particles can interfere with the venipuncture procedure
d) Because fasting increases the concentration of glucose in the blood

Answer: b) Because eating triggers the release of hormones that can affect glucose levels. Explanation: Eating triggers the release of insulin, a hormone that helps regulate glucose levels. To get an accurate measure of a patient's baseline glucose level, the patient is typically asked to fast before the test.

313. What role do platelets play in the body?
a) They carry oxygen
b) They fight infection
c) They initiate the clotting process
d) They regulate blood pH

Answer: c) They initiate the clotting process. Explanation: Platelets are cell fragments in the blood that stick together to initiate the clotting process when a blood vessel is injured. They play a crucial role in preventing excessive bleeding.

314. Why is the median cubital vein often the first choice for venipuncture?
a) It is the largest vein in the arm
b) It is the most superficial vein
c) It is well anchored and less likely to roll
d) It is the least painful to puncture

Answer: c) It is well anchored and less likely to roll. Explanation: The median cubital vein is often chosen for venipuncture because it is well anchored and less likely to roll, making it a more stable and reliable choice for blood draw.

315. Which of the following conditions would make a site unsuitable for venipuncture?
a) The vein is hard or cord-like
b) The vein is close to the surface of the skin
c) The vein is large and well anchored
d) The vein is easily palpable

Answer: a) The vein is hard or cord-like. Explanation: If a vein feels hard or cord-like, it may be sclerosed, or scarred, making it unsuitable for venipuncture. This is often a result of previous trauma or frequent venipuncture.

316. Why should you avoid drawing blood from an arm on the same side as a mastectomy without lymph nodes?
a) The blood draw can lead to lymphedema
b) The vein may be scarred from surgery
c) The patient may experience discomfort
d) All of the above

Answer: d) All of the above. Explanation: Drawing blood from the same side as a mastectomy without lymph nodes can lead to lymphedema, discomfort, and may be complicated by scarring from surgery.

317. What is the primary risk associated with choosing a hematoma as a site for venipuncture?
a) It will be more painful for the patient
b) It will cause the blood to hemolyze
c) It may lead to inaccurate test results
d) All of the above

Answer: d) All of the above. Explanation: A hematoma can cause pain for the patient, potentially cause the blood to hemolyze, and may result in inaccurate test results due to the mixture of tissue fluid with the blood sample.

318. Why is it important to clean the venipuncture site with an antiseptic?
a) To make the vein more visible
b) To reduce discomfort during venipuncture
c) To remove microorganisms and reduce risk of infection
d) To reduce bleeding after the venipuncture

Answer: c) To remove microorganisms and reduce risk of infection. Explanation: Cleaning the venipuncture site with an antiseptic helps to remove any surface microorganisms, reducing the risk of infection during and after the procedure.

319. Why should a phlebotomist avoid using a site where the vein crosses over a joint?
a) The vein is more likely to roll
b) The vein is less stable due to movement of the joint
c) The procedure can cause discomfort due to the sensitivity of the joint area
d) All of the above

Answer: d) All of the above. Explanation: Veins that cross over joints are less stable due to the movement of the joint, more likely to roll, and can cause more discomfort due to the sensitivity of the joint area.

320. Which vein is typically the last choice for venipuncture in the antecubital area?
a) Median cubital vein
b) Cephalic vein
c) Basilic vein
d) Metacarpal vein

Answer: c) Basilic vein. Explanation: The basilic vein is typically the last choice for venipuncture in the antecubital area because it is near the brachial artery and the median nerve, which can increase the risk of complications during the procedure.

321. What should be the direction of the needle during venipuncture?
a) Perpendicular to the vein
b) At a 45-degree angle to the vein
c) In line with the vein
d) Against the direction of blood flow

Answer: c) In line with the vein. Explanation: The needle should be inserted in line with the vein, typically at a 15 to 30 degree angle, to avoid going through the vein or causing trauma to the vein.

322. Why is it important to allow the antiseptic to air dry before venipuncture?
a) To ensure the complete removal of microorganisms
b) To reduce discomfort from the cold antiseptic
c) To avoid hemolysis of the blood sample
d) To prevent contamination of the blood sample with the antiseptic

Answer: d) To prevent contamination of the blood sample with the antiseptic. Explanation: Allowing the antiseptic to air dry ensures that it does not contaminate the blood sample, which could interfere with laboratory tests.

323. Why should you avoid venipuncture in an arm with a cannula or fistula for dialysis?
a) The procedure can damage the cannula or fistula
b) The procedure can lead to infection
c) The blood sample can be contaminated with dialysis fluid
d) All of the above

Answer: d) All of the above. Explanation: Venipuncture in an arm with a cannula or fistula for dialysis can damage the medical device, increase the risk of infection, and potentially contaminate the blood sample with dialysis fluid, interfering with laboratory tests.

324. You are performing a venipuncture on a patient with well-visible and palpable veins in both arms. However, the patient informs you that they had a mastectomy without lymph nodes on the right side. What should be your course of action?
a) Proceed with venipuncture on the right arm as it's visibly easier.
b) Perform venipuncture on the left arm.
c) Cancel the procedure.
d) Ask the patient which arm they would prefer for venipuncture.

Answer: b) Perform venipuncture on the left arm. Explanation: When a patient has undergone a mastectomy without lymph nodes, it's recommended to avoid venipuncture on that side due to risks like lymphedema, discomfort, and scarring complications.

325. During a venipuncture procedure, you encounter a vein that feels hard and cord-like upon palpation. What should be your next step?
a) Proceed with the venipuncture, as the vein's size will provide a good blood flow.
b) Choose a different site for venipuncture.
c) Apply a warm compress to soften the vein.
d) Ask the patient if this site has been used for venipuncture previously.

Answer: b) Choose a different site for venipuncture. Explanation: A hard, cord-like vein may be sclerosed or scarred and is not a suitable choice for venipuncture as it can cause discomfort to the patient and potential complications.

326. In a busy hospital setting, a patient's antecubital fossa area is the only accessible site, but there's a noticeable hematoma. What should be your approach?
a) Use the area with the hematoma, as it's the only accessible site.
b) Choose a site proximal to the hematoma for venipuncture.
c) Apply pressure to the hematoma to reduce it before proceeding.
d) Cancel the procedure as it's not safe.

Answer: b) Choose a site proximal to the hematoma for venipuncture. Explanation: Performing venipuncture on a hematoma can cause patient discomfort, increase the risk of hemolysis and lead to inaccurate test results.

327. While preparing for a venipuncture procedure, why should you allow the antiseptic to fully dry before proceeding?
a) To ensure all surface microbes are killed.
b) To make the skin less slippery.
c) To ensure the antiseptic does not dilute the blood sample.
d) To prevent a stinging sensation when the needle is inserted.

Answer: c) To ensure the antiseptic does not dilute the blood sample. Explanation: If the antiseptic is not completely dry, it could potentially contaminate and dilute the blood sample, leading to inaccurate test results.

328. When drawing blood from a patient with a dialysis fistula in their left arm, where would be the most suitable site for venipuncture?
a) In the right arm
b) In the left arm, but away from the fistula
c) Either arm, as long as you avoid the fistula
d) In the leg

Answer: a) In the right arm. Explanation: It's recommended to avoid venipuncture in an arm with a fistula for dialysis. Doing so can risk damage to the fistula, increase the risk of infection, and potentially contaminate the blood sample with dialysis fluid.

329. During a routine blood draw, you notice that the patient's vein appears to cross over a joint. What should you do?
a) Proceed with the venipuncture as the vein is clearly visible.
b) Apply a tourniquet to stabilize the vein.
c) Select another venipuncture site.
d) Ask the patient to hold their arm in a way that the vein doesn't cross the joint.

Answer: c) Select another venipuncture site. Explanation: You should avoid performing venipuncture across joints if possible. Movement of the joint could dislodge the needle, causing a hematoma or altering the blood sample.

330. While performing a venipuncture procedure on a dehydrated patient, you are unable to locate a suitable vein. What's the best course of action?
a) Ask the patient to drink water and return later.
b) Try using a smaller needle.
c) Attempt venipuncture on the patient's foot.
d) Apply a warm compress to the venipuncture site.

Answer: d) Apply a warm compress to the venipuncture site. Explanation: A warm compress can help dilate the veins, making them more visible and easier to puncture, especially in dehydrated patients.

331. During a blood draw, you notice a patient starting to faint. What should be your immediate response?
a) Continue the draw quickly so you can attend to the patient.
b) Stop the draw, remove the tourniquet, and ask the patient to put their head down.
c) Ask the patient to take deep breaths while you finish the draw.
d) Call for medical assistance and continue the draw.

Answer: b) Stop the draw, remove the tourniquet, and ask the patient to put their head down. Explanation: The patient's wellbeing is paramount. If a patient shows signs of fainting, you should immediately stop the draw and take appropriate measures to ensure their safety.

332. You are performing a venipuncture procedure on an elderly patient who has fragile, thin skin. What would be the best needle gauge to use?
a) 16-gauge needle
b) 18-gauge needle
c) 21-gauge needle
d) 23-gauge needle

Answer: d) 23-gauge needle. Explanation: Smaller gauge needles are ideal for patients with fragile veins as they are less likely to cause trauma or discomfort. In this case, a 23-gauge needle would be most appropriate.

333. When drawing blood for multiple routine tests, the order in which you fill the tubes is critical to prevent cross-contamination of additives between tubes. Which of the following is the correct order of draw?
a) Coagulation tube, EDTA tube, Serum tube
b) EDTA tube, Serum tube, Coagulation tube
c) Serum tube, Coagulation tube, EDTA tube
d) Coagulation tube, Serum tube, EDTA tube

Answer: a) Coagulation tube, EDTA tube, Serum tube. Explanation: The order of draw is important to avoid cross-contamination and maintain the integrity of the samples. The general order recommended by CLSI guidelines is: blood culture tubes, coagulation tubes (light blue), serum tubes with or without clot activator/gel (red, gold, or orange), heparin tubes (green), EDTA tubes (lavender), and then other additive tubes.

334. You are tasked with drawing a blood sample from a patient for a fasting blood glucose test. What is the most important question to ask before beginning the procedure?
a) "Have you had any water this morning?"
b) "Have you had any food or drink other than water in the last 8 hours?"
c) "Are you afraid of needles?"
d) "Do you feel comfortable with the venipuncture procedure?"

Answer: b) "Have you had any food or drink other than water in the last 8 hours?" Explanation: For a fasting blood glucose test, it's crucial that the patient has not had any caloric intake for at least 8 hours prior to the blood draw to ensure accurate results.

335. During a blood draw, the patient begins to have a vasovagal response. What immediate action should you take?
a) Complete the draw as quickly as possible.
b) Have the patient lay down and elevate their feet.
c) Immediately remove the needle and apply pressure to the site.
d) Inform the patient that the draw is almost complete and they will be fine.

Answer: c) Immediately remove the needle and apply pressure to the site. Explanation: Patient safety is the first priority. During a vasovagal response, it's important to immediately stop the draw, remove the needle, and apply pressure to the venipuncture site. After that, the patient should be positioned appropriately and monitored until they recover.

336. Which tube should be drawn first in a routine blood collection for the following tests: CBC, PT, and BMP?
a) Light blue top
b) Lavender top
c) Green top
d) Red top

Answer: a) Light blue top. Explanation: Following the order of draw, the light blue top (coagulation tube - PT test) should be drawn first, followed by the lavender top (hematology - CBC test), and lastly, the green or red top (chemistry - BMP test).

337. If a patient's vein collapses during a blood draw, what is the appropriate next step?
a) Continue drawing blood, the vein may reopen.
b) Reattempt the draw in a vein close to the collapsed one.
c) Apply a warm compress and try the draw again.
d) Remove the needle and choose a different puncture site.

Answer: d) Remove the needle and choose a different puncture site. Explanation: If a vein collapses during a draw, the procedure should be stopped. The needle should be removed, and another puncture site should be selected for a new attempt.

338. When collecting a routine blood specimen, how should the patient's arm be positioned?
a) Elevated above the heart
b) Lower than the heart
c) At heart level
d) Position doesn't affect the blood draw

Answer: b) Lower than the heart. Explanation: The patient's arm should be positioned comfortably with the forearm supported and the veins below the heart level. This promotes blood flow into the veins and makes them easier to visualize and palpate.

339. A patient appears anxious before a blood draw. Which of the following is an appropriate way to help ease their anxiety?
a) Rush through the procedure to minimize the time they have to worry
b) Ignore their anxiety and perform the draw as usual
c) Explain the procedure step by step and reassure them
d) Tell them to "toughen up" because it won't hurt that much

Answer: c) Explain the procedure step by step and reassure them. Explanation: Acknowledging the patient's anxiety and taking the time to explain the procedure can help alleviate fears. Good communication is an essential part of patient care.

340. You've been asked to collect a routine blood sample from an infant. Where would be the most appropriate site for collection?
a) The antecubital area of the arm
b) The dorsal hand veins
c) The heel
d) The radial artery

Answer: c) The heel. Explanation: For infants, the heel is often the best place to collect a blood sample. This is because the veins in the arms and hands are too small and fragile for venipuncture.

341. After a routine blood draw, a patient's puncture site continues to bleed. What is the most appropriate action to take?
a) Apply more pressure and elevate the arm.
b) Bandage the site tightly to stop the bleeding.
c) Reinsert the needle to clot the blood.
d) Ask the patient to apply pressure while you get help.

Answer: a) Apply more pressure and elevate the arm. Explanation: Continued bleeding can often be managed by applying more pressure to the site and elevating the arm above heart level. If bleeding continues, medical assistance should be sought.

342. What is the first step a phlebotomist should take in preparing for a venipuncture procedure?
a) Selecting the appropriate needle
b) Applying a tourniquet to the patient's arm
c) Patient identification and pre-examination process
d) Cleaning the puncture site

Answer: c) Patient identification and pre-examination process. Explanation: The first step in any medical procedure is always correctly identifying the patient and making sure they understand and consent to the procedure. This prevents any mix-ups and ensures the patient's safety.

343. When selecting the appropriate needle for a venipuncture, what aspect of the needle is not a determining factor?
a) Needle length
b) Needle gauge
c) Needle color
d) The bevel of the needle

Answer: c) Needle color. Explanation: The color of a needle doesn't determine its suitability for a venipuncture. The length, gauge, and the bevel of the needle are the factors that matter most.

344. The tourniquet is applied to a patient's arm during venipuncture in order to:
a) Comfort the patient
b) Prevent bleeding
c) Help visualize and palpate the veins
d) Cleanse the puncture site

Answer: c) Help visualize and palpate the veins. Explanation: A tourniquet is used to help visualize and palpate the veins by restricting the flow of blood.

345. The venipuncture site should be cleansed in what type of motion?
a) Up and down
b) Random circular motions
c) From the center outward in a spiral motion
d) Zig-zag motion

Answer: c) From the center outward in a spiral motion. Explanation: Cleaning the venipuncture site should begin at the center and move outward in a spiral motion. This reduces the likelihood of contaminants being moved toward the puncture site.

346. When collecting multiple samples during a venipuncture procedure, what determines the order in which the tubes are filled?
a) The volume of blood needed for each test
b) The color of the stoppers on the tubes
c) The type of additive in the tube
d) The size of the tubes

Answer: c) The type of additive in the tube. Explanation: The order of draw is determined by the type of additive in the tube. This prevents cross-contamination of additives between tubes.

347. Why should the phlebotomist release the tourniquet before withdrawing the needle during a venipuncture?
a) It minimizes discomfort to the patient.
b) It reduces the risk of hemolysis.
c) It prevents a hematoma.
d) All of the above.

Answer: d) All of the above. Explanation: Releasing the tourniquet before removing the needle reduces patient discomfort, decreases the risk of hemolysis (destruction of red blood cells), and helps prevent the formation of a hematoma.

348. What is the correct angle for needle insertion during a venipuncture?
a) 90 degrees
b) 45 degrees
c) 30 degrees
d) 15 degrees

Answer: c) 30 degrees. Explanation: The needle should be inserted at about a 30-degree angle. However, the angle can be adjusted to be shallower depending on the depth of the vein.

349. In a venipuncture procedure, what is the next step after the needle has been successfully inserted into the vein?
a) The tourniquet is released.
b) The first tube is attached to the needle holder.
c) The puncture site is cleaned.
d) The patient is asked to make a fist.

Answer: b) The first tube is attached to the needle holder. Explanation: After the needle is successfully inserted into the vein, the first collection tube is attached to the needle holder. This tube will fill with blood by vacuum.

350. Which of the following would be considered a reason to discontinue a venipuncture procedure immediately?
a) The patient becomes faint or nauseous.
b) The phlebotomist cannot locate a suitable vein.
c) The patient requests for the procedure to stop.
d) All of the above.

Answer: d) All of the above. Explanation: Patient safety and comfort are paramount. If a patient becomes unwell, if the phlebotomist cannot safely collect the sample, or if the patient requests the procedure to stop, it should be discontinued immediately.

351. After a venipuncture, the patient's puncture site continues to bleed. What should the phlebotomist do?
a) Clean the site with alcohol.
b) Apply a bandage immediately.
c) Reinsert the needle.
d) Apply pressure and elevate the arm.

Answer: d) Apply pressure and elevate the arm. Explanation: The most appropriate action is to apply pressure to the site and elevate the arm. This helps to slow the bleeding and encourages clotting.

352. You're performing a venipuncture on a patient and the vein collapses. What should you do next?
a) Continue with the draw, as the vein may still produce sufficient blood.
b) Apply a warm compress to the area.
c) Choose a new venipuncture site and start over.
d) Cancel the draw and reschedule the patient.

Answer: c) Choose a new venipuncture site and start over. Explanation: If a vein collapses during venipuncture, the correct response is to select a new site and restart the procedure. Continuing with the current site might not yield enough blood and can cause the patient discomfort.

353. During a routine blood collection, a patient faints. Which of the following actions should you take first?
a) Finish collecting the blood quickly.
b) Lay the patient down and elevate their legs.
c) Inform the patient's physician immediately.
d) Stop the blood collection and remove the tourniquet and needle.

Answer: d) Stop the blood collection and remove the tourniquet and needle. Explanation: Patient safety is always the priority. If a patient faints, the blood draw should be stopped immediately, and the tourniquet and needle removed.

354. You are collecting multiple tubes of blood from a patient. Which color tube should you fill first?
a) Red top
b) Lavender top
c) Green top
d) Gray top

Answer: a) Red top. Explanation: The recommended order of draw starts with blood culture bottles or tubes (yellow top), followed by coagulation tubes (light blue top). The red top tubes, which are non-additive tubes, come next.

355. A patient is exhibiting signs of anxiety before a venipuncture procedure. What strategy can you use to help calm their nerves?
a) Explain the procedure in detail, including possible complications.
b) Encourage them to look away and not focus on the procedure.
c) Tell them to think about something they find relaxing.
d) All of the above.

Answer: d) All of the above. Explanation: Each patient is different, and different strategies work for different people. All of the above strategies may help to calm a nervous patient.

356. You are about to perform a venipuncture on a patient who has had a mastectomy on her left side. What should you do?
a) Perform the venipuncture on the right arm.
b) Perform the venipuncture on the left arm.
c) Perform the venipuncture on either arm, but use a smaller needle.
d) Ask the patient which arm she prefers.

Answer: a) Perform the venipuncture on the right arm. Explanation: In patients who've had a mastectomy, it's recommended to avoid venipunctures on the side of the mastectomy due to risk of lymphedema.

357. In order to properly mix a blood sample with an additive in a collection tube, you should:
a) Shake the tube vigorously.
b) Turn the tube upside down 8-10 times.
c) Stir the tube with a clean needle.
d) Spin the tube in a centrifuge.

Answer: b) Turn the tube upside down 8-10 times. Explanation: Turning the tube gently upside down 8-10 times helps to mix the blood with the additive without causing hemolysis.

358. You've just completed a venipuncture and the patient's puncture site is still bleeding after 5 minutes. What is your best course of action?
a) Apply more pressure and continue to wait.
b) Call the patient's doctor immediately.
c) Bandage the site tightly to stop the bleeding.
d) Remove the bandage and check the site for a hematoma.

Answer: a) Apply more pressure and continue to wait. Explanation: In some cases, particularly with patients on anticoagulant medications, bleeding may take longer to stop. Continue applying pressure and reassess the site periodically.

359. While performing a venipuncture, a patient begins to have a seizure. Which of the following should you do first?
a) Continue the draw while another staff member assists the patient.
b) Remove the needle and tourniquet and move any sharp objects away from the patient.
c) Call for medical help immediately.
d) Try to restrain the patient to prevent injury.

Answer: b) Remove the needle and tourniquet and move any sharp objects away from the patient. Explanation: The immediate priority in this situation is patient safety. Remove the needle and tourniquet and ensure the patient's environment is safe.

360. You're performing a blood draw on a patient with difficult veins. You've already attempted the draw twice with no success. What should you do next?
a) Try one more time in a new location.
b) Ask a colleague for assistance.
c) Use a butterfly needle instead.
d) Cancel the draw and reschedule the patient.

Answer: b) Ask a colleague for assistance. Explanation: If two attempts have already been made without success, it's best to seek assistance from a more experienced colleague if possible. This is in the best interest of patient safety and comfort.

361. A patient's vein collapses during a venipuncture. What should be your immediate course of action?
a) Apply more pressure to the vein.
b) Try another vein in the same arm.
c) Proceed with the draw as the vein might recover.
d) Stop the procedure and remove the needle.

Answer: d) Stop the procedure and remove the needle. Explanation: In the case of a vein collapsing, the procedure should be stopped, the needle should be removed, and a new site should be chosen to prevent any discomfort or injury to the patient.

362. You notice a hematoma forming during the venipuncture. What should you do?
a) Release the tourniquet and stop the draw.
b) Apply more pressure to the area.
c) Try to draw from a different vein.
d) Continue the draw to finish quickly.

Answer: a) Release the tourniquet and stop the draw. Explanation: Hematoma formation indicates that blood has leaked into the tissue surrounding the venipuncture site. You should immediately stop the draw, release the tourniquet, and remove the needle.

363. During a routine blood draw, the patient begins to feel faint and nauseous. What should be your first response?
a) Continue the draw quickly, so you can lay the patient down.
b) Inform a supervisor immediately.
c) Stop the blood draw, and lay the patient down, if possible.
d) Ask the patient to take deep breaths and continue the draw.

Answer: c) Stop the blood draw, and lay the patient down, if possible. Explanation: If a patient begins to feel faint or nauseous, it's important to stop the blood draw immediately. The patient should be laid down, if possible, or asked to lower their head between their knees if they can't lay down.

364. During a venipuncture, the patient's vein starts to spasm. What should you do?
a) Continue with the draw, as spasms usually resolve on their own.
b) Pull the needle out slightly to relieve the spasm.
c) Try a different vein.
d) Stop the draw, remove the needle, and attempt the draw at another site.

Answer: d) Stop the draw, remove the needle, and attempt the draw at another site. Explanation: If a patient's vein begins to spasm, it can cause discomfort and potentially lead to a failed draw. In such a situation, it's best to stop the draw, remove the needle, and attempt the draw at a different site.

365. A patient has a known history of syncope (fainting) during blood draws. What precautionary measure should you take?
a) Have the patient lay down for the blood draw.
b) Ensure that you draw the blood as quickly as possible.
c) Have a colleague present in case the patient faints.
d) Avoid drawing blood from this patient.

Answer: a) Have the patient lay down for the blood draw. Explanation: For patients with a known history of fainting during blood draws, having them lay down during the procedure can help prevent a fainting episode.

366. After performing a venipuncture, the puncture site continues to bleed heavily. What should you do?
a) Bandage the site and ask the patient to keep the arm elevated.
b) Apply continuous pressure to the site for several minutes.
c) Perform another venipuncture at a different site.
d) Ask the patient to apply pressure while you seek help.

Answer: b) Apply continuous pressure to the site for several minutes. Explanation: In case of excessive bleeding post-venipuncture, you should apply continuous pressure to the site for several minutes until the bleeding stops. If the bleeding doesn't stop, seek medical help.

367. A patient starts to experience a severe allergic reaction during a blood draw. What should you do first?
a) Administer an antihistamine.
b) Call for immediate medical assistance.
c) Continue the blood draw as quickly as possible.
d) Ask the patient to take deep breaths to calm down.

Answer: b) Call for immediate medical assistance. Explanation: In case of a severe allergic reaction (anaphylaxis), immediate medical assistance is required. Continuing the blood draw or trying to calm the patient isn't appropriate in this situation.

368. You notice a patient's vein puncture site becoming increasingly swollen during the blood draw. What is the likely reason, and what should you do?
a) The vein has been punctured through, causing a hematoma; stop the blood draw and apply pressure to the site.
b) The tourniquet is too tight; loosen it and continue the draw.
c) The patient is having an allergic reaction; stop the draw and seek immediate medical assistance.
d) The needle is too large for the vein; stop the draw and choose a smaller needle.

Answer: a) The vein has been punctured through, causing a hematoma; stop the blood draw and apply pressure to the site. Explanation: If the puncture site is swelling, it's likely due to a hematoma caused by the vein being punctured through. The procedure should be stopped and pressure applied to the site to prevent further swelling and discomfort.

369. If your first attempt at venipuncture is unsuccessful, what should your initial action be?
a) Reassure the patient and prepare for a second attempt.
b) Apologize to the patient and stop the procedure.
c) Attempt the venipuncture in the same location.
d) Immediately call for a more experienced colleague.

Answer: a) Reassure the patient and prepare for a second attempt. Explanation: If the first attempt fails, you should reassure the patient, ensuring their comfort, and prepare for a second attempt. You should select a new venipuncture site and not attempt in the same location again.

370. In case of an unsuccessful venipuncture attempt, which of the following is not a recommended course of action?
a) Apologize to the patient for any discomfort caused.
b) Immediately try again in the same vein.
c) Reassess your technique and make necessary adjustments.
d) Prepare for another attempt, choosing a new venipuncture site.

Answer: b) Immediately try again in the same vein. Explanation: It is not recommended to try again in the same vein after a failed attempt, as this can increase the risk of complications. Instead, a new site should be chosen for the next attempt.

371. A patient is visibly upset after a failed venipuncture attempt. How should you respond?
a) Explain to the patient that this happens often.
b) Apologize and reassure the patient before attempting again.
c) Tell the patient to calm down so you can try again.
d) Inform the patient that they may need to seek care elsewhere.

Answer: b) Apologize and reassure the patient before attempting again. Explanation: It's important to acknowledge the patient's feelings, apologize for any discomfort caused, and reassure them before attempting the procedure again. Maintaining a calm, supportive demeanor can help alleviate the patient's concerns.

372. After a failed venipuncture attempt, the patient requests for a different phlebotomist. How should you handle this situation?
a) Insist on performing the venipuncture yourself to gain practice.
b) Respect the patient's wishes and arrange for a different phlebotomist.
c) Try to convince the patient that you can successfully perform the venipuncture.
d) Inform the patient that it's not possible to switch phlebotomists.

Answer: b) Respect the patient's wishes and arrange for a different phlebotomist. Explanation: Patient comfort and trust are paramount in medical procedures. If a patient requests a different phlebotomist, their wishes should be respected.

373. You have made a second unsuccessful attempt at venipuncture. What is the appropriate next step?
a) Make a third attempt.
b) Ask the patient to return another day.
c) Refer the patient to a specialist.
d) Ask a more experienced colleague for assistance.

Answer: d) Ask a more experienced colleague for assistance. Explanation: After two unsuccessful attempts, it is advised to seek help from a more experienced colleague. This helps ensure the patient's comfort and safety, as well as increases the chances of a successful venipuncture.

374. Following a failed venipuncture attempt, you notice the patient's puncture site becoming swollen and discolored. What should your immediate action be?
a) Continue with a second attempt.
b) Apply a bandage and ask the patient to keep an eye on it.
c) Apply pressure to the site and elevate the arm.
d) Ask a colleague to attempt the venipuncture.

Answer: c) Apply pressure to the site and elevate the arm. Explanation: Swelling and discoloration at the puncture site may indicate a hematoma. Applying pressure to the site and elevating the arm can help to prevent further blood leakage into the tissues.

375. After an unsuccessful venipuncture, the patient reports feeling faint. Which of the following steps should you take?
a) Have the patient lie down and raise their legs.
b) Ask the patient to leave and come back when they feel better.
c) Call for medical assistance.
d) Offer the patient some water and let them rest.

Answer: a) Have the patient lie down and raise their legs. Explanation: If a patient reports feeling faint after a failed venipuncture, it is crucial to have them lie down and raise their legs. This helps restore blood flow to the brain and may prevent a fainting episode.

376. After a failed venipuncture attempt, you notice that the puncture site continues to bleed despite pressure being applied. What should you do next?
a) Continue applying pressure and raise the patient's arm.
b) Clean the site and apply a new bandage.
c) Proceed with a second venipuncture attempt.
d) Refer the patient to their primary care provider.

Answer: a) Continue applying pressure and raise the patient's arm. Explanation: If the puncture site continues to bleed, you should continue to apply pressure and raise the patient's arm above the level of their heart. This will help slow the bleeding. If bleeding doesn't stop after several minutes, seek medical assistance.

377. You are unable to locate a suitable vein after a failed venipuncture attempt. What should you do next?
a) Try again in the same location.
b) Try a different location on the same arm.
c) Ask the patient to return another day.
d) Attempt venipuncture in the patient's foot.

Answer: b) Try a different location on the same arm. Explanation: If a suitable vein can't be located after a failed attempt, you should try a different location on the same arm. If unsuccessful, it may be necessary to try the other arm. Phlebotomists should be cautious about attempting venipuncture in the foot, as this should generally be avoided unless absolutely necessary and with a doctor's permission.

378. In which of the following cases would a capillary puncture be preferred over a venipuncture?
a) When large volumes of blood are required for testing.
b) When the patient has good vein visibility and condition.
c) When the patient is severely dehydrated.
d) When testing requires only a small volume of blood.

Answer: d) When testing requires only a small volume of blood. Explanation: Capillary puncture is typically used when only a small volume of blood is needed for the test. It's also beneficial for patients with difficult veins or for pediatric patients.

379. When performing a capillary puncture, what is the first line of action after cleaning the puncture site?
a) Apply a bandage to the puncture site.
b) Puncture the skin with a lancet.
c) Massage the area to increase blood flow.
d) Allow the site to air dry.

Answer: d) Allow the site to air dry. Explanation: After cleaning the puncture site with alcohol, you must allow it to air dry before proceeding to prevent hemolysis and avoid contaminating the sample.

380. In a capillary puncture, the first drop of blood is typically:
a) Discarded.
b) Immediately applied to the test strip or slide.
c) Used for glucose testing.
d) Saved for further testing.

Answer: a) Discarded. Explanation: The first drop of blood is usually discarded because it may contain tissue fluid, which could dilute the sample and potentially affect test results.

381. Why is it not recommended to use the thumb or index finger for capillary puncture?
a) These fingers have a slower blood flow.
b) The thumb and index finger are more sensitive to pain.
c) There is a higher risk of infection in these fingers.
d) It is more difficult to control a lancet on these fingers.

Answer: b) The thumb and index finger are more sensitive to pain. Explanation: The thumb and index finger are generally more sensitive to pain due to a higher concentration of nerve endings, which can make the procedure more uncomfortable for the patient.

382. The depth of a lancet puncture in capillary blood collection should not exceed:
a) 1.0 mm.
b) 2.0 mm.
c) 3.0 mm.
d) 5.0 mm.

Answer: b) 2.0 mm. Explanation: For capillary punctures, the depth of the puncture should typically not exceed 2.0 mm to avoid damaging deeper tissues and causing unnecessary pain.

383. What type of patients is capillary puncture often preferred for?
a) Elderly patients with visible veins.
b) Patients needing large volumes of blood drawn.
c) Patients with a fear of needles.
d) Neonates and small children.

Answer: d) Neonates and small children. Explanation: Capillary puncture is often preferred for neonates and small children because it's less invasive and requires a smaller blood volume than venipuncture.

384. When performing a capillary puncture, why is it important not to "milk" the finger too hard?
a) It may cause the patient discomfort.
b) It can lead to contamination of the sample with tissue fluids.
c) It can cause the blood to clot.
d) It might damage the lancet.

Answer: b) It can lead to contamination of the sample with tissue fluids. Explanation: Milking the finger too hard can cause tissue fluid to mix with the blood sample, which could dilute the sample and lead to inaccurate test results.

385. Which part of the body is the best site for a capillary puncture in adults?
a) The tip of the index finger.
b) The heel.
c) The distal segment of the ring finger.
d) The earlobe.

Answer: c) The distal segment of the ring finger. Explanation: For adults, the ring finger is generally the best site for a capillary puncture because it is less sensitive and has a sufficient capillary network.

386. Which of the following would be a reason NOT to perform a capillary puncture?
a) The patient has cold hands.
b) The patient has an infection in the finger.
c) The patient has good veins.
d) The test only requires a small amount of blood.

Answer: b) The patient has an infection in the finger. Explanation: If a patient has an infection in the finger, a capillary puncture should not be performed due to the risk of spreading the infection.

387. In performing a capillary puncture, what is the correct angle for the lancet to penetrate the skin?
a) Perpendicular to the fingerprint lines.
b) Parallel to the fingerprint lines.
c) At a 45-degree angle to the fingerprint lines.
d) At a 90-degree angle to the finger.

Answer: a) Perpendicular to the fingerprint lines. Explanation: When performing a capillary puncture, the lancet should penetrate the skin perpendicular to the fingerprint lines. This allows for a cleaner puncture and helps avoid slicing through the skin.

388. What should be the first step when preparing for a capillary puncture?
a) Apply the tourniquet.
b) Clean the site with an alcohol swab.
c) Collect all the necessary supplies.
d) Warm the puncture site.

Answer: c) Collect all the necessary supplies. Explanation: Before starting the procedure, it's crucial to ensure that all the necessary supplies - including gloves, lancets, microcontainers, and alcohol swabs - are at hand.

389. After cleaning the site for a capillary puncture with an alcohol swab, what is the next step?
a) Warm the puncture site.
b) Wait for the site to air dry.
c) Immediately puncture the site with a lancet.
d) Put on gloves.

Answer: b) Wait for the site to air dry. Explanation: After cleaning the site with an alcohol swab, it's crucial to let it air dry to prevent stinging or burning during the puncture, and to ensure the sample isn't contaminated by the alcohol.

390. Which of the following pieces of equipment is NOT necessary for a capillary puncture?
a) Microcontainer
b) Lancet
c) Tourniquet
d) Alcohol swabs

Answer: c) Tourniquet. Explanation: While a tourniquet is commonly used in venipuncture to make veins more prominent, it's not typically used in capillary puncture procedures.

391. What is the appropriate depth for a lancet puncture in a capillary blood collection for an adult?
a) 0.5 to 1.0 mm
b) 1.0 to 2.0 mm
c) 2.0 to 3.0 mm
d) 3.0 to 4.0 mm

Answer: b) 1.0 to 2.0 mm. Explanation: For capillary punctures in adults, the depth of the puncture should typically be 1.0 to 2.0 mm to avoid damaging deeper tissues and causing unnecessary pain.

392. Which of the following is the primary piece of equipment used to pierce the skin in a capillary puncture?
a) Syringe
b) Butterfly needle
c) Scalpel
d) Lancet

Answer: d) Lancet. Explanation: A lancet is the primary tool used to make a quick, clean puncture in the skin for capillary blood collection.

393. Once a capillary puncture has been performed, what should be done with the first drop of blood?
a) Discard it.
b) Collect it in a microcontainer.
c) Use it for testing.
d) Wipe it off with an alcohol swab.

Answer: a) Discard it. Explanation: The first drop of blood is usually discarded as it might be contaminated with tissue fluid, which could potentially affect the accuracy of test results.

394. What should a phlebotomist do if blood flow stops during a capillary puncture?
a) Apply more pressure with the lancet.
b) Perform another puncture immediately next to the first one.
c) Gently massage the puncture site to stimulate blood flow.
d) Abandon the procedure and try again later.

Answer: c) Gently massage the puncture site to stimulate blood flow. Explanation: If blood flow stops or slows during a capillary puncture, the phlebotomist can gently massage the area near the puncture site (not the site itself) to encourage blood flow. However, care should be taken not to "milk" the site too vigorously, as this can lead to contamination of the sample with tissue fluid.

395. How should a phlebotomist handle the patient's finger after a capillary puncture?
a) Apply a bandage.
b) Clean the puncture site with an alcohol swab.
c) Leave it alone to air dry.
d) Elevate the patient's hand.

Answer: a) Apply a bandage. Explanation: After a capillary puncture, the phlebotomist should apply a bandage to the puncture site to stop bleeding and protect the wound.

396. Where should a phlebotomist dispose of a used lancet after a capillary puncture?
a) In the regular trash.
b) In a biohazard waste bag.
c) In a sharps container.
d) In a designated container for used lancets.

Answer: c) In a sharps container. Explanation: After use, a lancet should be immediately placed in a sharps container to prevent accidental injuries and exposure to bloodborne pathogens.

397. After completing a capillary puncture, in what order should the phlebotomist do the following tasks: remove gloves, label the sample, dispose of the lancet, apply a bandage?
a) Dispose of the lancet, apply a bandage, remove gloves, label the sample.
b) Apply a bandage, dispose of the lancet, remove gloves, label the sample.
c) Apply a bandage, dispose of the lancet, label the sample, remove gloves.
d) Dispose of the lancet, remove gloves, apply a bandage, label the sample.

Answer: c) Apply a bandage, dispose of the lancet, label the sample, remove gloves. Explanation: The order of these tasks is crucial to ensure safety and accurate test results. After applying a bandage to the puncture site, the lancet should be disposed of in a sharps container. Then, still wearing gloves, the phlebotomist should label the sample to ensure its traceability. Only after these tasks are completed should the gloves be removed.

398. If a patient reports feeling faint during a capillary puncture procedure, what should the phlebotomist do?
a) Continue the procedure as quickly as possible.
b) Ask the patient to lay down and elevate their feet.
c) Have the patient drink a glass of water.
d) Dismiss the patient's complaint as nerves.

Answer: b) Ask the patient to lay down and elevate their feet. Explanation: Fainting or feeling lightheaded is a common response to blood draw procedures. Laying down and elevating the feet can help increase blood flow to the brain and potentially prevent a fainting episode.

399. When performing a capillary puncture on an infant, which site should generally be avoided?
a) The finger.
b) The earlobe.
c) The heel.
d) The toe.

Answer: a) The finger. Explanation: In infants, the heel is the preferred site for capillary punctures. Fingers should generally be avoided due to their small size and the risk of injury.

400. What precautionary measure can be taken to prevent bruising at the capillary puncture site?
a) Applying a bandage immediately after the puncture.
b) Applying pressure to the puncture site after blood collection.
c) Warming the puncture site prior to blood collection.
d) Cleaning the puncture site thoroughly before the puncture.

Answer: b) Applying pressure to the puncture site after blood collection. Explanation: Applying pressure to the puncture site immediately after blood collection can help to stop bleeding and prevent bruising.

401. What is the most appropriate action for a phlebotomist to take if a capillary puncture yields inadequate blood flow for collection?
a) Continue pressing the lancet into the puncture site.
b) Perform another puncture immediately next to the first one.
c) Gently massage or warm the area to stimulate blood flow.
d) Ask the patient to squeeze their hand repeatedly.

Answer: c) Gently massage or warm the area to stimulate blood flow. Explanation: Massaging or warming the area can help to stimulate blood flow and yield a better sample. The other options could lead to injury or contamination of the sample.

402. Which of the following complications is most likely if a capillary puncture is performed too deeply?
a) Hemolysis of the blood sample.
b) Inadequate blood flow.
c) Contamination of the blood sample.
d) Bone injury or infection.

Answer: d) Bone injury or infection. Explanation: If the puncture is too deep, especially in infants or elderly patients, there's a risk of injuring the bone or introducing infection.

403. Which technique can help prevent contamination of the blood sample during a capillary puncture?
a) Applying an antiseptic to the puncture site after the procedure.
b) Discarding the first drop of blood.
c) Using a larger lancet to ensure adequate blood flow.
d) Asking the patient to wash their hands prior to the procedure.

Answer: b) Discarding the first drop of blood. Explanation: The first drop of blood may be contaminated with tissue fluid or cleaning agent, which could potentially affect the accuracy of test results.

404. What is the most appropriate response if a patient develops a hematoma during a capillary puncture procedure?
a) Apply a cold compress to the area.
b) Continue the procedure to collect enough blood.
c) Reattempt the puncture on the other side of the same finger.
d) Immediately refer the patient to a physician.

Answer: a) Apply a cold compress to the area. Explanation: If a hematoma develops, the procedure should be stopped. Applying a cold compress can help to reduce swelling and discomfort.

405. How should a phlebotomist handle a patient who is uncooperative during a capillary puncture procedure?
a) Proceed with the procedure regardless of the patient's behavior.
b) Use physical restraint to ensure the patient stays still.
c) Try to reassure and calm the patient, or involve a caregiver if available.
d) Cancel the procedure and refer the patient to a more experienced colleague.

Answer: c) Try to reassure and calm the patient, or involve a caregiver if available. Explanation: Patient comfort and cooperation are crucial for a successful and safe procedure. If a patient is uncooperative, the phlebotomist should try to calm them down, explain the procedure, and involve a caregiver if possible.

406. Which of the following is NOT a suitable action to take if a patient experiences pain during a capillary puncture?
a) Stop the procedure immediately.
b) Reassure the patient that the pain is normal.
c) Try a different puncture site.
d) Reduce the depth of the puncture.

Answer: b) Reassure the patient that the pain is normal. Explanation: While some discomfort can be expected during a capillary puncture, significant pain is not normal and should be addressed by stopping the procedure, attempting a different puncture site, or adjusting technique.

407. When should a phlebotomist use a butterfly needle for capillary puncture?
a) When the patient is afraid of needles.
b) When the patient is dehydrated.
c) When the patient's veins are difficult to access.
d) Butterfly needles should not be used for capillary puncture.

Answer: d) Butterfly needles should not be used for capillary puncture. Explanation: Butterfly needles are typically used for venipuncture, not capillary puncture. For capillary puncture, a lancet is typically used to puncture the skin and draw blood.

408. Which action should be taken immediately after withdrawing the needle from a venipuncture procedure?
a) Apply an adhesive bandage to the puncture site.
b) Instruct the patient to raise their arm above their head.
c) Clean the puncture site with an antiseptic wipe.
d) Apply pressure to the puncture site.

Answer: d) Apply pressure to the puncture site. Explanation: Applying pressure immediately after withdrawing the needle helps to stop bleeding and minimize bruising.

409. If a patient begins to faint during the aftercare of a venipuncture procedure, what should the phlebotomist do?
a) Continue with the aftercare procedure as the faint feeling will pass.
b) Position the patient in the Trendelenburg position, if possible.
c) Instruct the patient to take deep breaths while standing.
d) Give the patient a glass of water and ask them to drink it quickly.

Answer: b) Position the patient in the Trendelenburg position, if possible. Explanation: If a patient feels faint or dizzy, laying them down and elevating their feet (Trendelenburg position) can help blood flow to the brain and prevent loss of consciousness.

410. Which is NOT part of standard aftercare following a venipuncture procedure?
a) Instructing the patient to keep the bandage on for at least 24 hours.
b) Providing information about potential complications.
c) Asking the patient to flex and extend their arm to stop bleeding.
d) Observing the patient for signs of adverse reactions.

Answer: c) Asking the patient to flex and extend their arm to stop bleeding. Explanation: Flexing and extending the arm after venipuncture could increase bleeding or bruising. Pressure should be applied to stop bleeding, and then a bandage applied.

411. What is an appropriate step to take for a patient who has experienced a hematoma after a venipuncture procedure?
a) Advise the patient to apply a warm compress to the area.
b) Instruct the patient to elevate the arm for 24 hours.
c) Advise the patient to apply a cold compress to the area.
d) Instruct the patient to avoid any physical activity for 48 hours.

Answer: c) Advise the patient to apply a cold compress to the area. Explanation: Applying a cold compress can reduce swelling and discomfort associated with a hematoma.

412. After a capillary puncture procedure, the patient complains of continued bleeding from the puncture site. What should the phlebotomist do?
a) Advise the patient to wash the area with soap and water.
b) Apply an additional adhesive bandage without removing the original.
c) Advise the patient to return to the medical facility immediately.
d) Instruct the patient to apply additional pressure to the puncture site.

Answer: d) Instruct the patient to apply additional pressure to the puncture site. Explanation: Additional pressure can help stop the bleeding. If bleeding continues despite pressure, the patient may need to return to the medical facility.

413. In general, how long should pressure be applied to a venipuncture site after needle withdrawal to help prevent bruising and bleeding?
a) At least 2 minutes.
b) Until the bleeding stops.
c) At least 5 minutes.
d) Until the patient feels comfortable.

Answer: b) Until the bleeding stops. Explanation: The length of time can vary, but pressure should be applied until bleeding has stopped. This helps prevent bruising and continued bleeding.

414. After a venipuncture procedure, when should the patient be instructed to remove the bandage?
a) Immediately when they get home.
b) After 24 hours.
c) When the bleeding has completely stopped.
d) After 3-4 hours.

Answer: b) After 24 hours. Explanation: Keeping the bandage on for about 24 hours helps to protect the puncture site and prevent infection.

415. Which of the following is NOT a sign of an adverse reaction to a venipuncture procedure during aftercare monitoring?
a) Increased heart rate
b) Feeling of warmth at the puncture site
c) Discoloration around the puncture site
d) Reduced pulse rate

Answer: d) Reduced pulse rate. Explanation: A reduced pulse rate is not typically associated with adverse reactions to a venipuncture procedure. Increased heart rate, warmth, and discoloration could suggest an infection or other complication.

416. What is the best course of action if a patient complains of numbness in the arm following a venipuncture procedure?
a) Advise the patient to perform arm exercises to restore feeling.
b) Advise the patient to apply a cold compress to the site.
c) Advise the patient to apply a warm compress to the site.
d) Advise the patient to seek immediate medical attention.

Answer: d) Advise the patient to seek immediate medical attention. Explanation: Numbness could be a sign of nerve damage or other serious complications, and should be evaluated by a healthcare provider immediately.

417. In what circumstance is it appropriate to remove the bandage from a venipuncture site earlier than instructed?
a) If the bandage becomes saturated with blood.
b) If the patient wants to shower or bathe.
c) If the bandage becomes uncomfortable.
d) It is never appropriate to remove the bandage early.

Answer: a) If the bandage becomes saturated with blood. Explanation: A saturated bandage could indicate continued bleeding and should be replaced. However, the patient should also seek medical attention if bleeding continues.

418. Used needles should be disposed of in which of the following?
a) Regular trash bin
b) Red biohazard bag
c) Sharps container
d) Recycling bin

Answer: c) Sharps container. Explanation: Needles and other sharp objects should always be disposed of in a sharps container to prevent needlestick injuries and potential transmission of infections.

419. What is the main risk associated with improper disposal of used phlebotomy equipment?
a) Equipment damage
b) Fire hazard
c) Patient confidentiality breach
d) Needlestick injuries and infection transmission

Answer: d) Needlestick injuries and infection transmission. Explanation: Improperly disposed needles can cause injuries and potentially transmit infections like Hepatitis and HIV.

420. Which is NOT a step in mitigating risks associated with improper disposal of phlebotomy equipment?
a) Re-capping needles before disposal
b) Using a sharps container
c) Training staff on proper disposal procedures
d) Regularly replacing full sharps containers

Answer: a) Re-capping needles before disposal. Explanation: Needles should never be recapped before disposal, as this increases the risk of a needlestick injury.

421. In the event of a needlestick injury, what should the affected healthcare worker do FIRST?
a) Wash the area with soap and water
b) Report the incident to their supervisor
c) Apply a bandage to the wound
d) Administer first aid to themselves

Answer: a) Wash the area with soap and water. Explanation: The immediate step is to wash the area to reduce the risk of infection. Then the incident should be reported and appropriate follow-up care sought.

422. What is one of the consequences of not replacing a sharps container when it is three-quarters full?
a) It can lead to cross-contamination.
b) It can result in needlestick injuries.
c) It is more likely to spill.
d) It can lead to equipment failure.

Answer: b) It can result in needlestick injuries. Explanation: Overfilled sharps containers increase the risk of needlestick injuries as needles can protrude from the opening.

423. If a phlebotomist observes a colleague improperly disposing of used equipment, what should they do?
a) Ignore it if it's a one-time occurrence.
b) Confront the colleague and correct them.
c) Report the incident to a supervisor.
d) Dispose of the equipment properly themselves.

Answer: c) Report the incident to a supervisor. Explanation: It's important to maintain a safe environment. Reporting the incident ensures the issue can be addressed and proper training can be provided if necessary.

424. Which of the following is NOT a part of proper phlebotomy equipment disposal?
a) Disposing of gloves in a regular trash bin.
b) Immediately disposing of used needles in a sharps container.
c) Discarding blood tubes in a regular trash bin.
d) Disposing of used gauze in a biohazard bag.

Answer: c) Discarding blood tubes in a regular trash bin. Explanation: Blood tubes may contain residual blood and should be disposed of as biohazardous waste, not in regular trash.

425. If a sharps container is not available, what should be done with used needles?
a) Place them in a sturdy, plastic container until a sharps container is available.
b) Place them in a biohazard bag until a sharps container is available.
c) Dispose of them in a regular trash bin.
d) Keep them on the phlebotomy tray until a sharps container is available.

Answer: a) Place them in a sturdy, plastic container until a sharps container is available. Explanation: If a sharps container is not available, a sturdy, plastic container can provide temporary storage, but used needles should be transferred to a sharps container as soon as possible.

426. Which of the following is NOT a consequence of improper disposal of used phlebotomy equipment?
a) Environmental pollution.
b) Risk of fire.
c) Transmission of infectious diseases.
d) Needlestick injuries.

Answer: b) Risk of fire. Explanation: Improper disposal of phlebotomy equipment mainly raises concerns of needlestick injuries and infection transmission, not a fire risk.

427. Who is responsible for the proper disposal of used phlebotomy equipment?
a) The phlebotomist who used the equipment.
b) The patient on whom the equipment was used.
c) The healthcare facility's cleaning staff.
d) Any staff member present during the procedure.

Answer: a) The phlebotomist who used the equipment. Explanation: The person who uses the equipment, in this case the phlebotomist, is typically responsible for its safe disposal.

428. Which of the following is the best practice for blood sample handling immediately after collection?
a) Keep the sample at room temperature until processing.
b) Put the sample in a freezer as soon as possible.
c) Immediately expose the sample to direct sunlight.
d) Gently invert the sample to mix additives.

Answer: d) Gently invert the sample to mix additives. Explanation: Most blood collection tubes contain additives that must be mixed with the blood sample. Gently inverting the tube immediately after collection ensures this.

429. What is the primary risk associated with storing blood samples at inappropriate temperatures?
a) Degradation of sample quality.
b) Over coagulation of the sample.
c) It may cause discomfort to the patient.
d) The sample may spill.

Answer: a) Degradation of sample quality. Explanation: Incorrect storage temperatures can degrade the quality of the sample, potentially altering test results.

430. What should be done immediately after a blood sample is drawn?
a) It should be stored in a refrigerator.
b) It should be processed for testing.
c) It should be labeled with patient information.
d) It should be disposed of properly.

Answer: c) It should be labeled with patient information. Explanation: It is essential to label the blood sample immediately after collection to ensure proper patient identification and prevent mix-ups.

431. What is the best way to ensure the integrity of a blood sample during transportation?
a) Transport the sample in a cooler with ice.
b) Ensure the sample is transported as quickly as possible.
c) Keep the sample in a sealed biohazard bag.
d) Expose the sample to heat to maintain viscosity.

Answer: c) Keep the sample in a sealed biohazard bag. Explanation: Transporting the sample in a sealed biohazard bag helps to protect it from contamination and maintain its integrity.

432. Why should a phlebotomist avoid shaking a blood sample?
a) It can cause hemolysis.
b) It can mix the blood with other samples.
c) It can disrupt the coagulation process.
d) It can cause the patient discomfort.

Answer: a) It can cause hemolysis. Explanation: Shaking a blood sample can lead to hemolysis or breaking of red blood cells, which can affect test results.

433. What is the primary purpose of centrifuging a blood sample?
a) To heat the sample.
b) To mix the sample.
c) To separate components of the sample.
d) To cool the sample.

Answer: c) To separate components of the sample. Explanation: Centrifugation separates blood components based on their densities, which is often required for certain types of testing.

434. Which of the following information is NOT required when labeling a blood sample?
a) Patient's full name.
b) Date and time of collection.
c) Phlebotomist's name.
d) The temperature at the time of collection.

Answer: d) The temperature at the time of collection. Explanation: The temperature at the time of collection is not typically required on a blood sample label.

435. If a blood sample needs to be refrigerated, what is the general guideline for the temperature range?
a) 2-8 degrees Celsius.
b) 10-15 degrees Celsius.
c) 20-25 degrees Celsius.
d) 30-35 degrees Celsius.

Answer: a) 2-8 degrees Celsius. Explanation: Generally, refrigeration for blood samples is typically done at a temperature range of 2-8 degrees Celsius.

436. Which of the following would be the best practice when storing a blood sample that does not require refrigeration?
a) Store the sample in direct sunlight.
b) Keep the sample in a cool, dark place.
c) Store the sample near a heat source.
d) Keep the sample in a place with high humidity.

Answer: b) Keep the sample in a cool, dark place. Explanation: For samples that do not require refrigeration, it's best to store them in a cool, dark place to prevent degradation.

437. A serum separator tube (SST) has been filled with a blood sample. What is the next step?
a) The tube should be inverted 5-6 times and allowed to clot for 30 minutes.
b) The tube should be placed directly in the refrigerator.
c) The sample should be immediately centrifuged.
d) The tube should be shaken vigorously.

Answer: a) The tube should be inverted 5-6 times and allowed to clot for 30 minutes. Explanation: SSTs are designed to facilitate blood clotting. Inverting the tube helps mix the clot activator with the blood, and allowing it to sit aids in clot formation before centrifugation.

438. In the event of a patient experiencing an adverse reaction post-venipuncture, what should be the first step taken by a phlebotomist?
a) Contacting the family members of the patient.
b) Immediately reporting to their supervisor.
c) Assisting the patient and ensuring their immediate safety.
d) Documenting the incident in the patient's chart.

Answer: c) Assisting the patient and ensuring their immediate safety. Explanation: The first step in any adverse event is always patient safety.

439. Upon noticing a post-procedure complication in a patient, when should the phlebotomist document the incident?
a) Immediately, without attending to the patient.
b) After providing necessary care to the patient.
c) After discussing with colleagues.
d) At the end of their shift.

Answer: b) After providing necessary care to the patient. Explanation: Although documentation is important, it should never be prioritized over patient care.

440. Who should a phlebotomist report to in case of an adverse event or complications post-venipuncture or post-capillary puncture?
a) The patient's primary care physician.
b) The charge nurse or immediate supervisor.
c) The hospital CEO.
d) The patient's family.

Answer: b) The charge nurse or immediate supervisor. Explanation: In most medical settings, the charge nurse or the immediate supervisor should be the first to know about any adverse events or complications.

441. What details are most crucial when documenting an adverse event post-venipuncture?
a) The patient's emotional state.
b) The time of the event and the actions taken.
c) The phlebotomist's personal feelings about the event.
d) Suggestions for preventing future similar events.

Answer: b) The time of the event and the actions taken. Explanation: The most critical aspects to document are the factual details of the event, including when it occurred and what actions were taken in response.

442. In case of a needlestick injury to the phlebotomist during venipuncture, what should be the immediate step taken?
a) Disinfect the area and apply a bandage.
b) Report to the immediate supervisor.
c) Continue with the procedure if the patient did not notice.
d) Go home and take rest.

Answer: a) Disinfect the area and apply a bandage. Explanation: The first step after a needlestick injury is to immediately disinfect the area and apply a bandage to prevent infection.

443. Where should the details of an adverse event following a venipuncture procedure be recorded?
a) In the patient's medical records.
b) In the phlebotomist's personal diary.
c) On a sticky note attached to the patient's file.
d) Verbally communicated to the next shift.

Answer: a) In the patient's medical records. Explanation: Documentation of adverse events should be made in the patient's medical records to maintain an official, accessible account of the incident.

444. In the case of a serious adverse event following venipuncture, such as syncope, which team should be immediately alerted?
a) The janitorial team.
b) The patient's family.
c) The Rapid Response Team.
d) The hospital management.

Answer: c) The Rapid Response Team. Explanation: The Rapid Response Team (or a similar emergency response team depending on the facility) is trained to quickly respond to serious medical situations.

445. After an adverse event, it is discovered that the phlebotomist did not follow the standard protocol during the procedure. What is likely to be the next step?
a) The phlebotomist will be immediately fired.
b) The incident will be discussed with the phlebotomist, and appropriate training will be provided.
c) The incident will be ignored since the patient is stable.
d) The phlebotomist will be asked to apologize to the patient.

Answer: b) The incident will be discussed with the phlebotomist, and appropriate training will be provided. Explanation: In most professional settings, if an error occurred due to a lapse in following protocol, the phlebotomist will receive additional training to prevent future incidents.

446. Which of the following is the most crucial factor in preventing future adverse events during venipuncture?
a) Following standard protocol for each procedure.
b) Having a supervisor present during each procedure.
c) Using high-quality needles and tubes.
d) Reassuring the patient that adverse events are rare.

Answer: a) Following standard protocol for each procedure. Explanation: While all these factors can contribute to safe procedures, consistently following standard protocol is the most important factor in preventing complications.

447. What is the primary purpose of a blood culture?
a) To check for the presence of microorganisms in the blood.
b) To determine the patient's blood type.
c) To measure cholesterol levels.
d) To assess the number of red blood cells.

Answer: a) To check for the presence of microorganisms in the blood. Explanation: Blood cultures are used primarily to detect the presence of bacteria or fungi in the blood.

448. Why is it important to collect multiple sets of blood cultures?
a) It increases the chance of detecting intermittent bacteremia.
b) It ensures that there is enough blood for testing.
c) It is a standard requirement for all patients.
d) It reduces the risk of contamination.

Answer: a) It increases the chance of detecting intermittent bacteremia. Explanation: Multiple sets of blood cultures increase the likelihood of capturing bacteria or fungi that may not constantly be present in the bloodstream.

449. How does blood culture collection differ from standard venipuncture?
a) The puncture site must be disinfected twice in blood culture collection.
b) Blood culture collection requires a larger needle.
c) Blood culture collection is typically performed on the foot.
d) Blood culture collection does not require a tourniquet.

Answer: a) The puncture site must be disinfected twice in blood culture collection. Explanation: The skin at the puncture site is typically disinfected twice in blood culture collection to reduce the risk of contamination.

450. What is the recommended order of draw for blood culture bottles?
a) Aerobic then anaerobic.
b) Anaerobic then aerobic.
c) It doesn't matter as long as both are collected.
d) The order of draw is not applicable to blood cultures.

Answer: a) Aerobic then anaerobic. Explanation: The recommended order of draw is to first collect the aerobic bottle, which encourages the growth of oxygen-using bacteria, and then the anaerobic bottle.

451. Which of the following is an indicator of a positive blood culture result?
a) The blood culture bottle remains clear.
b) The blood culture bottle turns green.
c) The blood culture bottle shows signs of cloudiness or color change.
d) The blood culture bottle explodes.

Answer: c) The blood culture bottle shows signs of cloudiness or color change. Explanation: Cloudiness or a color change in the blood culture bottle can indicate growth of microorganisms.

452. Why is the timing of blood culture collection critical in febrile patients?
a) To coincide with meal times.
b) To allow for immediate testing.
c) To capture bacteria or fungi during fever spikes.
d) To avoid patient discomfort.

Answer: c) To capture bacteria or fungi during fever spikes. Explanation: Blood cultures are often collected during fever spikes because bacteria or fungi may be more likely to be present in the bloodstream at this time.

453. What is the main concern with blood culture collections?
a) Patient discomfort.
b) Blood volume.
c) Contamination.
d) Cost.

Answer: c) Contamination. Explanation: Contamination of blood cultures can lead to false-positive results, which can result in unnecessary treatment.

454. Which of the following is NOT an appropriate site for blood culture collection?
a) Antecubital fossa.
b) Wrist.
c) Back of the hand.
d) Dorsal metacarpal veins.

Answer: b) Wrist. Explanation: The wrist is generally avoided for venipuncture due to the presence of nerves and tendons.

455. How should blood culture bottles be stored before being transported to the lab?
a) Refrigerated.
b) At room temperature.
c) Heated.
d) Frozen.

Answer: b) At room temperature. Explanation: Blood culture bottles should be stored at room temperature to promote the growth of microorganisms.

456. Why is it important to fill blood culture bottles to the recommended volume?
a) To ensure the bottle doesn't overflow.
b) To promote proper ratio of blood to media.
c) To prevent leakage during transport.
d) To ensure easy identification of the sample.

Answer: b) To promote proper ratio of blood to media. Explanation: Filling blood culture bottles to the recommended volume ensures an appropriate blood-to-media ratio, which increases the chance of detecting microorganisms.

457. Why should a phlebotomist wear gloves when collecting a blood culture?
a) To protect the patient from infection.
b) To protect the phlebotomist from infection.
c) To adhere to standard procedures.
d) All of the above.

Answer: d) All of the above. Explanation: Gloves act as a barrier, protecting both the patient and the phlebotomist from potential infection, and their use is a part of the standard protocol.

458. What is the first step in preparing a patient's arm for blood culture collection?
a) Apply a tourniquet.
b) Disinfect the puncture site.
c) Ask the patient to make a fist.
d) Find a suitable vein.

Answer: a) Apply a tourniquet. Explanation: The tourniquet is applied first to facilitate the vein becoming more visible and palpable.

459. How should the puncture site be disinfected before blood culture collection?
a) With soap and water.
b) With a standard alcohol swab.
c) With a chlorhexidine swab.
d) Disinfection is not necessary.

Answer: c) With a chlorhexidine swab. Explanation: Chlorhexidine is preferred for disinfecting the puncture site because it is more effective at killing bacteria than alcohol.

460. Why is the needle inserted with the bevel up during venipuncture for blood culture collection?
a) To ensure a smoother entry.
b) To minimize patient discomfort.
c) To minimize damage to the vein.
d) All of the above.

Answer: d) All of the above. Explanation: Inserting the needle with the bevel up can make entry smoother, lessen patient discomfort, and reduce potential damage to the vein.

461. What should a phlebotomist do if they suspect that a blood culture bottle has been contaminated?
a) Proceed with testing.
b) Discard the bottle and collect a new sample.
c) Send the bottle to the lab with a note about possible contamination.
d) Cleanse the bottle with an alcohol swab.

Answer: b) Discard the bottle and collect a new sample. Explanation: If there's any suspicion of contamination, it's crucial to start over to avoid a false-positive result.

462. Why is it important to fill the blood culture bottles to the correct volume?
a) To prevent spillage during transport.
b) To ensure an adequate sample for testing.
c) To maintain the correct blood-to-broth ratio.
d) To make the bottles easier to handle.

Answer: c) To maintain the correct blood-to-broth ratio. Explanation: Maintaining the correct blood-to-broth ratio in the culture bottles is key to promoting the growth of any bacteria or fungi present.

463. Which of the following is NOT an appropriate action after a blood culture collection?
a) Apply pressure to the puncture site.
b) Dispose of used needles in a regular trash bin.
c) Label the blood culture bottles at the patient's bedside.
d) Send the blood culture bottles to the lab promptly.

Answer: b) Dispose of used needles in a regular trash bin. Explanation: Used needles are considered biohazardous waste and should be disposed of in a designated sharps container.

464. Why is it important to collect blood cultures before starting antibiotic therapy?
a) Antibiotics can make the patient uncomfortable.
b) Antibiotics can interfere with the culture results.
c) Antibiotics can cause a false-positive result.
d) Antibiotics can change the color of the blood.

Answer: b) Antibiotics can interfere with the culture results. Explanation: Antibiotics can kill bacteria or inhibit their growth, potentially leading to a false-negative blood culture result.

465. Which of the following statements is true regarding the collection of multiple sets of blood cultures?
a) They are collected from the same vein.
b) They are collected to increase the likelihood of detecting bacteremia.
c) They are collected simultaneously.
d) They are collected using the same needle.

Answer: b) They are collected to increase the likelihood of detecting bacteremia. Explanation: Multiple sets of blood cultures are collected from separate venipuncture sites to increase the likelihood of detecting bacteremia.

466. Why should the blood culture bottles be incubated after collection?
a) To keep them at a safe temperature for transport.
b) To promote the growth of any microorganisms present.
c) To kill any microorganisms present.
d) To prepare them for disposal.

Answer: b) To promote the growth of any microorganisms present. Explanation: Incubating the blood culture bottles promotes the growth of any microorganisms present, which is necessary for accurate identification and sensitivity testing.

467. John, a 56-year-old male, has been instructed by his doctor to take an at-home glucose monitoring test due to his newly diagnosed diabetes. What advice would be most important to give to John?
a) He needs to fast for 12 hours before testing.
b) He should always clean the lancet after use.
c) He must ensure his hands are clean and dry before testing.
d) He needs to perform the test at the same time each day.

Answer: c) He must ensure his hands are clean and dry before testing. Explanation: For accurate results, John must ensure that his hands are clean and dry before performing the test. This is to prevent any residual substances on his fingers from interfering with the test results.

468. A phlebotomist has been asked to collect a stool sample from a patient suspected of having a gastrointestinal infection. Which of the following would be a critical instruction for the patient?
a) The stool sample should be mixed with urine.
b) The patient should use a laxative to speed up the process.
c) The stool sample should be free from toilet paper and water.
d) The patient should collect all stool passed in a 24-hour period.

Answer: c) The stool sample should be free from toilet paper and water. Explanation: To avoid contamination and inaccurate results, the stool sample should be free from foreign substances, including toilet paper and water.

469. A patient comes in for a therapeutic phlebotomy due to polycythemia vera. Which of the following is the primary consideration during the procedure?
a) The speed of blood draw should be faster than a standard draw.
b) The volume of blood to be removed should be based on patient symptoms.
c) Only the lightest gauge needle should be used.
d) The patient's vitals must be monitored during the procedure.

Answer: d) The patient's vitals must be monitored during the procedure. Explanation: Therapeutic phlebotomy can cause significant shifts in a patient's blood volume and pressure, so monitoring vitals throughout the procedure is crucial to ensure patient safety.

470. A pediatric patient requires a heel stick for a bilirubin test. What is the maximum depth for the heel puncture?
a) 1.0 mm
b) 2.0 mm
c) 2.4 mm
d) 3.0 mm

Answer: c) 2.4 mm. Explanation: For infants, the heel stick depth should not exceed 2.4 mm to prevent injury to the calcaneus, or heel bone.

471. A phlebotomist is preparing to perform a sweat chloride test on a 2-month-old baby suspected of having cystic fibrosis. How is the sweat sample collected for this test?
a) By having the baby exercise.
b) Using a special collection pad.
c) Via a heel stick.
d) Using a syringe to draw sweat.

Answer: b) Using a special collection pad. Explanation: For a sweat chloride test, sweat is induced on a small area of the skin using a process called iontophoresis. The sweat is then collected on a special pad or paper and analyzed for chloride content.

472. A phlebotomist is required to collect a blood sample for a peak level of a medication. When should this collection occur?
a) Immediately after the dose is administered.
b) Just before the next dose is due.
c) At the time specified by the medical professional.
d) Within an hour after the dose is administered.

Answer: c) At the time specified by the medical professional. Explanation: The timing of peak level sample collection can vary greatly depending on the medication. It should be collected at the time specified by the healthcare provider.

473. A patient needs to have a blood sample taken for a trough drug level. When should this sample be collected?
a) Just before the next dose is due.
b) Immediately after the dose is administered.
c) An hour after the dose is administered.
d) Two hours after the dose is administered.

Answer: a) Just before the next dose is due. Explanation: A trough level refers to the lowest concentration of a drug in the patient's bloodstream. Therefore, the blood sample should be taken just before the next dose is due.

474. A phlebotomist is performing a PKU test on a newborn. Which of the following is crucial to remember?
a) The baby should not be fed before the test.
b) The sample should be collected by a heel stick.
c) The test should be performed immediately after birth.
d) The baby's foot should be soaked in warm water before collection.

Answer: b) The sample should be collected by a heel stick. Explanation: A heel stick is the preferred method of blood collection for a PKU test in newborns. The other options are not standard procedures.

475. A phlebotomist is asked to collect a blood sample from a patient for an Ethanol test. Which of the following precautions should be followed?
a) The sample must be kept warm until testing.
b) The site must not be cleaned with an alcohol swab.
c) The patient must fast for 12 hours prior to testing.
d) The sample must be exposed to light before testing.

Answer: b) The site must not be cleaned with an alcohol swab. Explanation: Using an alcohol swab could contaminate the sample and result in a falsely elevated ethanol level. Instead, a non-alcohol antiseptic should be used to clean the puncture site.

476. A patient presents with symptoms of extreme thirst and frequent urination. The physician suspects diabetes and orders a glucose tolerance test (GTT). What is the first step in this procedure?
a) Ask the patient to consume a glucose solution immediately.
b) Perform a fasting blood sugar test.
c) Have the patient exercise vigorously.
d) Perform a random blood sugar test.

Answer: b) Perform a fasting blood sugar test. Explanation: The first step in a GTT is to establish a baseline by performing a fasting blood sugar test. This gives a reference point for how the patient's body manages glucose under normal conditions.

477. A pregnant woman is scheduled for a GTT to screen for gestational diabetes. How is the procedure performed?
a) The patient is asked to fast for 8 hours, then a fasting blood sample is drawn.
b) The patient is asked to consume a glucose solution immediately, then a fasting blood sample is drawn.
c) The patient is asked to consume a glucose solution, then a blood sample is drawn every hour for three hours.
d) The patient is asked to fast for 8 hours, then a blood sample is drawn every hour for three hours.

Answer: c) The patient is asked to consume a glucose solution, then a blood sample is drawn every hour for three hours. Explanation: In gestational diabetes screening, the patient consumes a glucose solution and blood samples are drawn at timed intervals to see how the body metabolizes the glucose.

478. A patient has been instructed to return for a three-hour glucose tolerance test after a one-hour screening test indicated potential gestational diabetes. Which of the following best describes the protocol for this test?
a) The patient consumes a glucose drink and blood samples are taken at one-hour intervals.
b) The patient fasts overnight and then blood samples are taken at one-hour intervals.
c) The patient fasts overnight, consumes a glucose drink, and blood samples are taken at one-hour intervals.
d) The patient does not need to fast but blood samples are taken at one-hour intervals.

Answer: c) The patient fasts overnight, consumes a glucose drink, and blood samples are taken at one-hour intervals. Explanation: The standard protocol for a three-hour GTT involves an overnight fast, then consumption of a glucose drink. Blood samples are taken at one-hour intervals to monitor how the body metabolizes the glucose.

479. The healthcare provider suspects reactive hypoglycemia in a patient. Which test is likely to be ordered?
a) Fasting glucose test.
b) Glucose tolerance test.
c) Hemoglobin A1c.
d) Random blood sugar test.

Answer: b) Glucose tolerance test. Explanation: A glucose tolerance test is used to diagnose reactive hypoglycemia. This condition is characterized by low blood sugar within a few hours after eating, so it's essential to monitor the patient's response to glucose over a period of time.

480. A patient has a strong family history of type 2 diabetes but currently shows no symptoms. What would a healthcare provider most likely order?
a) An immediate glucose tolerance test.
b) A fasting blood glucose test annually.
c) A glucose tolerance test annually.
d) Weekly random blood glucose tests.

Answer: b) A fasting blood glucose test annually. Explanation: For individuals at high risk but currently asymptomatic, it's typically recommended to perform a fasting blood glucose test annually, rather than a glucose tolerance test.

481. A phlebotomist is explaining the procedure for a GTT to a patient. Which of the following is important to mention?
a) The patient must refrain from physical activity during the test.
b) The patient can continue eating as normal during the test.
c) The patient must consume a glucose solution between each blood draw.
d) The patient can leave the clinic between blood draws.

Answer: a) The patient must refrain from physical activity during the test. Explanation: During a GTT, the patient should remain seated and avoid physical activity as it could affect the metabolism of glucose.

482. In a 2-hour glucose tolerance test, at what time points are blood samples typically collected?
a) Start of the test, 30 minutes, 1 hour, and 2 hours.
b) Start of the test and at 2 hours.
c) Start of the test, 1 hour, and 2 hours.
d) Start of the test and at 1 hour.

Answer: c) Start of the test, 1 hour, and 2 hours. Explanation: For a 2-hour GTT, blood samples are typically collected at the start (fasting), 1 hour, and 2 hours after the patient consumes the glucose solution.

483. A patient arrives for a glucose tolerance test but forgot to fast. What should the phlebotomist do?
a) Proceed with the test as planned.
b) Only perform the fasting blood glucose portion of the test.
c) Reschedule the test.
d) Ask the patient to fast in the waiting room for 2 hours before starting the test.

Answer: c) Reschedule the test. Explanation: It's crucial for the patient to fast before a GTT to ensure accurate results. If the patient has not fasted, the test should be rescheduled.

484. A phlebotomist notices that a patient appears dizzy and disoriented during a glucose tolerance test. What is the appropriate course of action?
a) Discontinue the test and alert a nurse or doctor.
b) Offer the patient a snack to increase their blood sugar.
c) Encourage the patient to lie down but continue with the test.
d) Continue the test as these are normal side effects of fasting.

Answer: a) Discontinue the test and alert a nurse or doctor. Explanation: If a patient becomes symptomatic during a GTT, such as experiencing dizziness or confusion, the test should be discontinued and a healthcare provider should be alerted immediately. This could indicate a serious issue like hypoglycemia.

485. After completing the initial fasting glucose test for a glucose tolerance test (GTT), what is the next step the phlebotomist should take?
a) Instruct the patient to consume a high-sugar meal.
b) Administer a glucose solution to the patient.
c) Collect a second blood sample immediately.
d) Send the patient home with instructions for a second fasting blood test.

Answer: b) Administer a glucose solution to the patient. Explanation: Following the fasting glucose test, the next step in a GTT is for the patient to consume a glucose solution. This allows the phlebotomist to evaluate how the patient's body metabolizes glucose over time.

486. A patient arrives for a GTT but admits to having eaten breakfast. What should the phlebotomist do?
a) Proceed with the test regardless.
b) Ask the patient to fast for the next two hours before starting the test.
c) Reschedule the test.
d) Perform only the fasting blood glucose portion of the test.

Answer: c) Reschedule the test. Explanation: The patient must be in a fasted state for the GTT to provide accurate results. If the patient has not fasted, the test should be rescheduled.

487. In a GTT, what is the typical timeframe for collecting blood samples after the patient has consumed the glucose solution?
a) Every 30 minutes for 2 hours.
b) Every hour for 2-3 hours.
c) Immediately after consumption and again at 2 hours.
d) Only after 2 hours.

Answer: b) Every hour for 2-3 hours. Explanation: In a standard GTT, blood samples are collected every hour for 2-3 hours after the patient consumes the glucose solution.

488. When preparing a glucose solution for a GTT, which of the following is important to consider?
a) The solution must be refrigerated before administration.
b) The solution must contain a specific concentration of glucose.
c) The solution must be flavored to make it more palatable for the patient.
d) The solution must be warmed before administration.

Answer: b) The solution must contain a specific concentration of glucose. Explanation: The glucose solution used for a GTT must contain a specific concentration of glucose, typically 75 grams for adults, to ensure accurate results.

489. During a GTT, a patient reports feeling faint and sweaty. What is the most appropriate course of action for the phlebotomist?
a) Continue with the test as these are common side effects.
b) Encourage the patient to lie down and rest, then continue with the test.
c) Immediately discontinue the test and notify a healthcare provider.
d) Administer a second dose of the glucose solution.

Answer: c) Immediately discontinue the test and notify a healthcare provider. Explanation: Symptoms such as faintness and sweating during a GTT may indicate hypoglycemia, a potentially dangerous condition. The test should be discontinued immediately and a healthcare provider should be notified.

490. What is therapeutic phlebotomy primarily used for?
a) Drawing small quantities of blood for laboratory testing.
b) Reducing blood volume to treat certain medical conditions.
c) Collecting blood for transfusions to other patients.
d) Administering medications via the bloodstream.

Answer: b) Reducing blood volume to treat certain medical conditions.
Explanation: Therapeutic phlebotomy is a procedure used to remove larger volumes of blood than typically taken during diagnostic testing to reduce blood volume or decrease levels of red blood cells or iron, which can help in treating certain medical conditions.

491. Polycythemia vera is a condition where there is an increased number of red blood cells in the blood. What role does therapeutic phlebotomy play in its management?
a) It decreases the number of white blood cells.
b) It reduces the number of red blood cells.
c) It increases the production of red blood cells.
d) It has no effect on the number of red blood cells.

Answer: b) It reduces the number of red blood cells.
Explanation: In patients with polycythemia vera, therapeutic phlebotomy is used to decrease the number of red blood cells, thereby reducing blood viscosity and the risk of clot formation.

492. What is the term for a disorder characterized by excessive iron absorption leading to iron overload, which can be treated with therapeutic phlebotomy?
a) Thalassemia
b) Iron-deficiency anemia
c) Hemochromatosis
d) Hemophilia

Answer: c) Hemochromatosis.
Explanation: Hemochromatosis is a condition characterized by excessive absorption and deposition of iron in the body. Therapeutic phlebotomy is one of the primary treatments, as it removes iron-rich blood from the body.

493. Which of the following is NOT a typical indication for therapeutic phlebotomy?
a) Chronic iron deficiency
b) Polycythemia vera
c) Hemochromatosis
d) Porphyria cutanea tarda

Answer: a) Chronic iron deficiency.
Explanation: Chronic iron deficiency would not be treated with therapeutic phlebotomy as this procedure removes blood and would exacerbate an iron deficiency. The other conditions listed are indications for therapeutic phlebotomy.

494. During therapeutic phlebotomy, how much blood is typically removed at one time?
a) 5-10 mL
b) 50-100 mL
c) 250-500 mL
d) 1-2 Liters

Answer: c) 250-500 mL
Explanation: Therapeutic phlebotomy usually involves removing larger volumes of blood than diagnostic testing, typically around 250-500 mL per session.

495. In what way should a patient be prepared for therapeutic phlebotomy?
a) By fasting for 12 hours prior to the procedure.
b) By drinking extra fluids prior to the procedure.
c) By refraining from taking any medications for 24 hours before the procedure.
d) By avoiding physical activity for 48 hours prior to the procedure.

Answer: b) By drinking extra fluids prior to the procedure.
Explanation: Encouraging the patient to drink extra fluids before therapeutic phlebotomy helps in maintaining proper hydration levels since a substantial volume of blood will be removed.

496. In therapeutic phlebotomy, blood letting should be conducted:
a) As quickly as possible.
b) Slowly, at a controlled rate.
c) In multiple small aliquots.
d) With the patient in a standing position.

Answer: b) Slowly, at a controlled rate.
Explanation: Blood letting in therapeutic phlebotomy should be conducted slowly and at a controlled rate to prevent hypotension and ensure patient stability.

497. What is the primary purpose of therapeutic phlebotomy?
a) To collect large quantities of blood for transfusion.
b) To remove excess iron from the body.
c) To reduce blood volume in the body.
d) To prepare the patient for major surgery.

Answer: c) To reduce blood volume in the body. Explanation: Therapeutic phlebotomy is often used to reduce the amount of blood in the body. This can help manage conditions where excess blood volume or constituents cause health problems.

498. Which of the following conditions might warrant therapeutic phlebotomy?
a) Anemia
b) Hemochromatosis
c) Hemophilia
d) Leukemia

Answer: b) Hemochromatosis. Explanation: Hemochromatosis is a condition characterized by excessive iron absorption, which can lead to iron overload. Therapeutic phlebotomy can help manage this condition by removing excess iron in the blood.

499. In the case of polycythemia vera, why is therapeutic phlebotomy performed?
a) To lower the patient's blood pressure.
b) To remove excess red blood cells.
c) To treat infection.
d) To manage pain.

Answer: b) To remove excess red blood cells. Explanation: Polycythemia vera is a condition that results in an abnormally high number of red blood cells. Therapeutic phlebotomy can help manage this condition by reducing the number of red blood cells.

500. When performing therapeutic phlebotomy, what type of equipment would a phlebotomist typically use?
a) Butterfly needle
b) Central venous catheter
c) Standard-sized needle
d) Large-bore needle

Answer: d) Large-bore needle. Explanation: Therapeutic phlebotomy often involves the removal of larger volumes of blood than routine blood draws. Therefore, a large-bore needle is typically used to accommodate the higher flow rates.

501. Which of the following is an essential step in pre-procedure planning for therapeutic phlebotomy?
a) Ensure the patient has fasted.
b) Confirm the patient's blood type.
c) Evaluate the patient's hydration status.
d) Check the patient's immunization records.

Answer: c) Evaluate the patient's hydration status. Explanation: Prior to therapeutic phlebotomy, the phlebotomist should evaluate the patient's hydration status. Dehydrated patients might require rehydration to safely tolerate the procedure.

502. During therapeutic phlebotomy, a patient starts to feel dizzy. What should the phlebotomist do?
a) Encourage the patient to drink water.
b) Stop the procedure and lower the patient's head.
c) Increase the rate of blood removal.
d) Ignore the symptoms, as they are common during this procedure.

Answer: b) Stop the procedure and lower the patient's head. Explanation: If a patient becomes dizzy during therapeutic phlebotomy, the procedure should be stopped and the patient's head should be lowered to increase blood flow to the brain. Medical assistance should be sought.

503. Therapeutic phlebotomy is typically indicated for treating which of the following conditions?
a) Thalassemia
b) Sickle cell anemia
c) Iron deficiency anemia
d) Leukemia

Answer: a) Thalassemia. Explanation: Thalassemia is a blood disorder in which the body produces an abnormal form of hemoglobin. This can lead to an excess of iron in the body. Therapeutic phlebotomy can help manage iron overload.

504. In a patient undergoing therapeutic phlebotomy, what is one potential risk to monitor for during the procedure?
a) Iron overload
b) Hemolysis
c) Hypovolemia
d) Blood clotting

Answer: c) Hypovolemia. Explanation: Hypovolemia, or low blood volume, can be a potential risk in therapeutic phlebotomy, particularly if large volumes of blood are removed. It's crucial to monitor the patient for signs of dizziness, fainting, or other symptoms of hypovolemia during and after the procedure.

505. Which of the following can be a long-term effect of frequent therapeutic phlebotomy procedures?
a) Decreased platelet count
b) Iron deficiency
c) High cholesterol levels
d) Increased white blood cell count

Answer: b) Iron deficiency. Explanation: Frequent therapeutic phlebotomy can potentially lead to iron deficiency over time, as the procedure involves removing blood (and therefore, iron) from the body.

506. How often is therapeutic phlebotomy typically performed in the treatment of hemochromatosis?
a) Once a week
b) Once a month
c) Every six months
d) Once a year

Answer: a) Once a week. Explanation: For the treatment of hemochromatosis, therapeutic phlebotomy is typically performed once a week until iron levels normalize. The frequency may be adjusted based on the patient's specific needs and response to treatment.

507. Which of the following is the first step in performing a therapeutic phlebotomy?
a) Secure the vein with a tourniquet.
b) Obtain a detailed medical history from the patient.
c) Clean the puncture site with an antiseptic.
d) Administer a local anesthetic to the puncture site.

Answer: b) Obtain a detailed medical history from the patient. Explanation: Prior to the procedure, the phlebotomist should review the patient's medical history and current medications, which can affect the procedure and potential outcomes.

508. What is the optimal position for a patient during a therapeutic phlebotomy procedure?
a) Standing
b) Sitting upright
c) Lying flat
d) Semi-reclining

Answer: d) Semi-reclining. Explanation: The patient should be in a semi-reclining position during the procedure. This position helps to prevent fainting and allows for easy intervention if the patient starts feeling unwell.

509. After the puncture site has been cleaned, what is the next step in therapeutic phlebotomy?
a) Apply pressure to the puncture site.
b) Insert the needle at a 30-degree angle.
c) Secure the vein with a tourniquet.
d) Attach the blood bag to the needle.

Answer: b) Insert the needle at a 30-degree angle. Explanation: The needle is inserted into the vein at a 30-degree angle to the skin, with the bevel facing upwards.

510. What should a phlebotomist do if a patient begins to feel faint during a therapeutic phlebotomy?
a) Encourage the patient to breathe deeply and slowly.
b) Stop the procedure immediately and lower the patient's head.
c) Offer the patient a snack to boost their blood sugar.
d) Continue with the procedure, as fainting is a common reaction.

Answer: b) Stop the procedure immediately and lower the patient's head. Explanation: If a patient feels faint during a therapeutic phlebotomy, the procedure should be stopped immediately. The patient's head should be lowered to increase blood flow to the brain.

511. Which of the following complications can arise from therapeutic phlebotomy?
a) Hyperkalemia
b) Hemolysis
c) Iron overload
d) Hypovolemia

Answer: d) Hypovolemia. Explanation: Hypovolemia, or low blood volume, can occur after therapeutic phlebotomy, particularly if large volumes of blood are removed. It's important to monitor the patient for signs of dizziness, fainting, or other symptoms of hypovolemia during and after the procedure.

512. What should a phlebotomist do following the removal of the needle from a therapeutic phlebotomy?
a) Apply pressure to the site with a sterile gauze.
b) Immediately bandage the puncture site.
c) Ask the patient to lift their arm above their head.
d) Discard the used needle into a sharps container.

Answer: a) Apply pressure to the site with a sterile gauze. Explanation: Direct pressure should be applied to the puncture site with a sterile gauze to stop bleeding. This should be done before bandaging the site and discarding the used needle.

513. Which type of needle is most commonly used for therapeutic phlebotomy?
a) Butterfly needle
b) 22-gauge needle
c) 16-gauge needle
d) Insulin needle

Answer: c) 16-gauge needle. Explanation: A 16-gauge needle is most commonly used for therapeutic phlebotomy due to the large volumes of blood that need to be removed during the procedure.

514. How is the blood flow rate controlled during therapeutic phlebotomy?
a) By adjusting the size of the needle.
b) By adjusting the position of the patient.
c) By adjusting the tourniquet pressure.
d) By adjusting the height of the blood bag.

Answer: d) By adjusting the height of the blood bag. Explanation: During therapeutic phlebotomy, the height of the blood bag is adjusted to control the rate of blood flow.

515. What is the maximum volume of blood typically removed during a single therapeutic phlebotomy procedure?
a) 250 mL
b) 500 mL
c) 750 mL
d) 1000 mL

Answer: b) 500 mL. Explanation: Typically, up to 500 mL of blood is removed during a single therapeutic phlebotomy session. However, this amount can vary depending on the patient's individual needs and condition.

516. Which of the following best defines Point of Care Testing (POCT)?
a) It refers to tests that are performed near a patient and at the site of patient care.
b) It is the process of collecting, transporting, and analyzing patient samples in a central laboratory.
c) It refers to advanced laboratory techniques performed only by clinical scientists.
d) It is a specific group of tests used to diagnose genetic diseases.

Answer: a) It refers to tests that are performed near a patient and at the site of patient care. Explanation: POCT is characterized by its convenience and speed, as it is performed close to the site of patient care, often by non-laboratory medical staff.

517. What is a significant benefit of POCT compared to traditional laboratory testing?
a) POCT always provides more accurate results.
b) POCT requires highly specialized training and skills.
c) POCT results can be available immediately, aiding in quick decision making.
d) POCT tests can only be conducted in large hospitals or laboratories.

Answer: c) POCT results can be available immediately, aiding in quick decision making. Explanation: One of the main advantages of POCT is that it provides immediate results, allowing for faster clinical decisions and improved patient care.

518. Which of the following is a challenge associated with POCT?
a) The tests are typically more expensive than traditional lab tests.
b) The results of POCT are never reliable.
c) All POCT procedures are invasive.
d) Only a limited number of tests can be performed using POCT.

Answer: a) The tests are typically more expensive than traditional lab tests. Explanation: While POCT provides convenience and speed, the tests are typically more expensive than their traditional laboratory counterparts.

519. How can the quality of POCT be ensured?
a) By not allowing any form of control testing or calibration.
b) By performing all POCT outside of a controlled laboratory environment.
c) Through regular training of personnel, use of control materials, and participation in external quality assurance programs.
d) By using the same standard laboratory equipment and protocols.

Answer: c) Through regular training of personnel, use of control materials, and participation in external quality assurance programs. Explanation: Quality assurance in POCT is crucial and can be achieved through regular training, quality control testing, and participation in external quality assurance programs.

520. Which of the following is not an advantage of POCT?
a) Rapid turnaround time for test results.
b) Enhanced patient satisfaction due to immediate feedback.
c) Lower cost compared to traditional lab tests.
d) Potential to improve patient outcomes by enabling quick clinical management decisions.

Answer: c) Lower cost compared to traditional lab tests. Explanation: While POCT offers numerous benefits such as quick results and improved patient satisfaction, the tests are often more expensive than traditional lab tests.

521. Which of the following healthcare settings is less likely to utilize POCT?
a) Emergency rooms
b) Intensive care units
c) Centralized hospital laboratories
d) General practitioners' clinics

Answer: c) Centralized hospital laboratories. Explanation: Centralized hospital laboratories typically perform traditional laboratory testing, while POCT is more common in immediate care settings like emergency rooms, ICUs, and GP clinics.

522. What is the primary driving factor for the utilization of POCT?
a) Desire to publish research papers
b) Need for immediate test results to make quick clinical decisions
c) Preference for less accurate test results
d) Desire to reduce the role of central laboratories

Answer: b) Need for immediate test results to make quick clinical decisions. Explanation: The primary driving factor for the use of POCT is the need for immediate test results, which can enable healthcare providers to make quick, informed clinical decisions.

523. Who is typically responsible for performing POCT?
a) Only trained phlebotomists
b) Any healthcare professional, with appropriate training
c) Only the treating physician or nurse
d) Only medical laboratory scientists

Answer: b) Any healthcare professional, with appropriate training. Explanation: POCT can be performed by a wide range of healthcare professionals, as long as they have received appropriate training.

524. Which of the following is an example of a common POCT?
a) Blood glucose monitoring
b) Microscopic examination of tissue samples
c) Chromosome analysis for genetic disorders
d) Hormone level measurement in a central lab

Answer: a) Blood glucose monitoring. Explanation: Blood glucose monitoring is a common example of POCT, as it can be performed at the bedside or in the field with immediate results.

525. What is an essential aspect to consider for the successful implementation of POCT?
a) Ensuring POCT is only performed by highly specialized staff
b) Making sure POCT is less expensive than traditional lab testing
c) Guaranteeing that POCT is conducted without quality control
d) Ensuring the quality and reliability of POCT through training, control testing, and external quality assurance

Answer: d) Ensuring the quality and reliability of POCT through training, control testing, and external quality assurance. Explanation: To successfully implement POCT, it is essential to ensure the quality and reliability of tests through personnel training, regular control testing, and participation in external quality assurance programs.

526. What is one primary responsibility of a phlebotomist during POCT?
a) Designing and developing new POCT devices
b) Delivering the collected samples to a centralized lab
c) Performing the tests and ensuring accurate results
d) Delegating all patient interaction to a nurse or doctor

Answer: c) Performing the tests and ensuring accurate results. Explanation: During POCT, the phlebotomist is responsible for correctly performing the tests and ensuring the results are accurate, which requires specific knowledge and skills.

527. Which additional skill is essential for a phlebotomist performing POCT?
a) Ability to design testing protocols
b) Skill in operating a scanning electron microscope
c) Proficiency in performing open-heart surgery
d) Competency in using and maintaining the testing device

Answer: d) Competency in using and maintaining the testing device. Explanation: A phlebotomist performing POCT must have competency in using and maintaining the testing device to ensure accurate and reliable results.

528. What is the primary equipment needed for glucose monitoring, a common POCT?
a) A computed tomography (CT) scanner
b) A blood glucose meter and test strips
c) A flow cytometer
d) An electron microscope

Answer: b) A blood glucose meter and test strips. Explanation: For glucose monitoring, a blood glucose meter and test strips are used. The meter measures the amount of glucose in a small sample of blood, usually drawn from pricking the patient's finger.

529. Which of the following is a standard technique in glucose monitoring POCT?
a) Collecting a venous blood sample and sending it to the laboratory
b) Pricking the patient's finger to get a small blood sample
c) Performing a surgical biopsy
d) Using a syringe to draw a large volume of blood

Answer: b) Pricking the patient's finger to get a small blood sample. Explanation: For glucose monitoring, a common technique is to prick the patient's finger with a small, sharp needle (lancet) to get a small blood sample, which is then tested with the blood glucose meter.

530. What is a common POCT used for coagulation testing?
a) Activated partial thromboplastin time (aPTT) test
b) Blood typing and crossmatching
c) Chromosome karyotyping
d) Complete blood count (CBC)

Answer: a) Activated partial thromboplastin time (aPTT) test. Explanation: The aPTT test, performed at the point of care, measures the time it takes for blood to clot. It is commonly used to monitor treatment with heparin, an anticoagulant medication.

531. For POCT coagulation testing, a phlebotomist typically uses:
a) A CT scanner
b) A coagulation analyzer
c) A cell counter
d) An electron microscope

Answer: b) A coagulation analyzer. Explanation: A coagulation analyzer is used for POCT coagulation tests. The device measures the time it takes for a clot to form in a blood sample, providing information about the body's ability to form clots.

532. Which of the following is an important consideration for a phlebotomist during POCT?
a) The phlebotomist should disregard quality control measures for speed
b) The phlebotomist should prioritize communication with the patient about the test results
c) The phlebotomist should conduct the test without prior patient consent
d) The phlebotomist should focus solely on collecting the sample and leave the analysis to the physicians

Answer: b) The phlebotomist should prioritize communication with the patient about the test results. Explanation: The phlebotomist should always prioritize effective communication with the patient, explaining the test results and answering any questions the patient may have, while maintaining strict adherence to confidentiality and privacy rules.

533. What should a phlebotomist do if a POCT result is outside the normal range?
a) Ignore it as the POCT devices are often unreliable
b) Contact the patient's primary healthcare provider immediately
c) Run the test again to double-check
d) Adjust the result to fall within the normal range

Answer: b) Contact the patient's primary healthcare provider immediately. Explanation: If a POCT result is outside the normal range, the phlebotomist should contact the patient's primary healthcare provider immediately so that appropriate action can be taken.

534. What is the role of a phlebotomist in maintaining the quality of POCT?
a) Phlebotomists are not involved in quality control for POCT
b) Phlebotomists should perform regular checks and control tests on POCT devices
c) Phlebotomists should clean the POCT devices once a year
d) Phlebotomists should delegate all quality control tasks to other healthcare professionals

Answer: b) Phlebotomists should perform regular checks and control tests on POCT devices. Explanation: Phlebotomists play an important role in maintaining the quality of POCT. This includes performing regular checks on the devices and conducting control tests to ensure the accuracy of the results.

535. What is one key quality control measure that phlebotomists should use in POCT to ensure accuracy and reliability?
a) Sending all tests to a central lab for verification
b) Routinely calibrating testing equipment
c) Ignoring the manufacturer's guidelines
d) Storing all test devices in a humid environment

Answer: b) Routinely calibrating testing equipment. Explanation: Calibration ensures that the testing equipment is working as expected and delivering accurate results. It is an essential quality control measure in POCT.

536. Which of the following is NOT a recommended quality control measure in POCT?
a) Following the manufacturer's instructions for use of test devices
b) Periodic calibration of test equipment
c) Testing the device with known samples
d) Modifying test procedures to expedite the process

Answer: d) Modifying test procedures to expedite the process. Explanation: All the other options represent important quality control measures. However, modifying test procedures to speed up the process can compromise the accuracy and reliability of the test results.

537. Why are control tests essential in POCT?
a) They help in training new phlebotomists
b) They help verify the accuracy and precision of the test
c) They substitute for patient samples in testing
d) They replace the need for calibration

Answer: b) They help verify the accuracy and precision of the test. Explanation: Control tests involve testing samples with known values to verify the accuracy and precision of the POCT device.

538. What is a critical step for a phlebotomist in documenting POCT results?
a) Omitting patient identification details for privacy
b) Recording the results in the patient's medical record
c) Disclosing the results to the patient's family
d) Ignoring any out-of-range results

Answer: b) Recording the results in the patient's medical record. Explanation: Accurate documentation of test results, including recording the results in the patient's medical record, is critical in patient care and for future reference.

539. Why is proper documentation of POCT results crucial in patient care?
a) It ensures all staff members have access to the patient's test results
b) It helps to bill the patient correctly
c) It is not crucial; it's just a formal requirement
d) It prevents the patient from knowing their results

Answer: a) It ensures all staff members have access to the patient's test results. Explanation: Proper documentation of POCT results is crucial as it ensures that all relevant staff members have access to the test results, which can inform diagnosis, treatment decisions, and ongoing management of the patient's condition.

540. When should a phlebotomist report POCT results?
a) Immediately after the test
b) After several days
c) Only when the results are within normal range
d) Only when the results are outside the normal range

Answer: a) Immediately after the test. Explanation: The results of a POCT should be reported immediately after the test so that any necessary medical interventions can be initiated without delay.

541. What should be included in the documentation of POCT results?
a) Patient identification, test results, date and time of test, and tester's identification
b) Only the patient's name and test results
c) Only the test results and date of test
d) The tester's identification and the test results

Answer: a) Patient identification, test results, date and time of test, and tester's identification. Explanation: Complete and accurate documentation of POCT results should include all the mentioned details to ensure traceability and accountability.

542. Who should a phlebotomist notify if a POCT result is outside the normal range?
a) The patient's family
b) The media
c) The patient's primary healthcare provider
d) The insurance company

Answer: c) The patient's primary healthcare provider. Explanation: If a POCT result is outside the normal range, the phlebotomist should contact the patient's primary healthcare provider immediately so that appropriate action can be taken.

543. If a POCT device fails a control test, what should a phlebotomist do?
a) Continue using the device, but document the failure
b) Report the failure and stop using the device until it's serviced
c) Run another test to confirm the failure
d) Ignore the failure since control tests are not always reliable

Answer: b) Report the failure and stop using the device until it's serviced. Explanation: If a POCT device fails a control test, the phlebotomist should stop using the device and report the failure. The device should be serviced before it is used again to ensure the accuracy of the results.

544. As a phlebotomist, which of the following practices can enhance the effectiveness of POCT?
a) Altering test procedures to make them faster
b) Providing patient education about the tests
c) Performing the tests without calibration
d) Ignoring quality control measures

Answer: b) Providing patient education about the tests. Explanation: Patient education can improve compliance, reduce anxiety, and contribute to better overall patient care, which in turn can improve the effectiveness of POCT.

545. In what way can a phlebotomist contribute to the improvement of POCT?
a) By ignoring any anomalies in test results
b) By ensuring that only calibrated equipment is used
c) By skipping the control tests for saving time
d) By not documenting the test results

Answer: b) By ensuring that only calibrated equipment is used. Explanation: Calibration is a crucial step in ensuring the accuracy of POCT results. By adhering to this practice, a phlebotomist can contribute to the improvement of POCT.

546. How can phlebotomists optimize the documentation process for POCT?
a) By using abbreviations that only they understand
b) By recording the test results immediately after performing the test
c) By skipping the documentation process for negative results
d) By not recording the date and time of the test

Answer: b) By recording the test results immediately after performing the test. Explanation: Timely documentation of POCT results can reduce errors and improve patient care.

547. Which of the following is NOT a way a phlebotomist can contribute to the optimization of POCT?
a) Regularly maintaining and checking equipment
b) Taking regular feedback from patients about their testing experience
c) Ignoring manufacturer's guidelines to save time
d) Continuing education to stay updated on new technologies and protocols

Answer: c) Ignoring manufacturer's guidelines to save time. Explanation: Ignoring manufacturer's guidelines can compromise the accuracy of test results and is not a recommended practice in POCT.

548. How can phlebotomists contribute to quality assurance in POCT?
a) By skipping the quality control tests
b) By performing tests on outdated machines
c) By incorporating control tests in their routine
d) By not reporting faulty machines

Answer: c) By incorporating control tests in their routine. Explanation: Quality control tests are an integral part of quality assurance in POCT. By incorporating these tests in their routine, phlebotomists can contribute to the overall quality of the testing process.

549. Which of the following actions can help a phlebotomist optimize patient comfort during POCT?
a) Performing tests without explaining the process to the patient
b) Using larger needles for drawing blood
c) Explaining the testing procedure and addressing any patient concerns
d) Rushing through the test to minimize the time the patient spends at the clinic

Answer: c) Explaining the testing procedure and addressing any patient concerns. Explanation: Taking the time to explain the testing procedure to the patient and addressing their concerns can enhance patient comfort and cooperation during POCT.

550. How can a phlebotomist enhance patient safety during POCT?
a) By ignoring standard hygiene practices
b) By following the guidelines for patient identification
c) By using the same needle for multiple patients
d) By not wearing any personal protective equipment

Answer: b) By following the guidelines for patient identification. Explanation: Proper patient identification is a critical aspect of patient safety in any testing procedure, including POCT.

551. What role can a phlebotomist play in optimizing the accuracy of POCT?
a) Ignoring calibration of equipment
b) Neglecting the manufacturer's instructions
c) Performing regular control tests
d) Not documenting any anomalies in test results

Answer: c) Performing regular control tests. Explanation: Regular control tests help ensure the accuracy of POCT by validating that the test equipment is functioning properly.

552. As a phlebotomist, what practice can improve the speed and efficiency of POCT without compromising accuracy?
a) Skipping quality control tests
b) Familiarizing oneself with the testing equipment and procedures
c) Ignoring calibration of the equipment
d) Not documenting the test results

Answer: b) Familiarizing oneself with the testing equipment and procedures. Explanation: Familiarity with the equipment and test procedures can significantly improve the speed and efficiency of POCT, without compromising on accuracy.

553. Which of the following is an incorrect practice for a phlebotomist aiming to optimize POCT?
a) Ignoring patient identification processes
b) Keeping up-to-date with advancements in POCT
c) Documenting test results accurately and timely
d) Participating in training and educational opportunities

Answer: a) Ignoring patient identification processes. Explanation: Correct patient identification is crucial for accurate POCT and patient safety. Ignoring this process can lead to errors and misdiagnosis.

554. What is the impact of improper specimen handling on test results in a clinical laboratory setting?
a) It can lead to inaccurate test results
b) It increases the speed of processing the tests
c) It has no impact on the test results
d) It improves the accuracy of the tests

Answer: a) It can lead to inaccurate test results. Explanation: Improper specimen handling can compromise the integrity of the specimen and result in inaccurate test results, affecting patient diagnosis and treatment.

556. Which of the following factors can compromise the integrity of collected specimens?
a) Properly timed specimen collection
b) Storage at appropriate temperatures
c) Prolonged exposure to light
d) Adequate labeling of specimens

Answer: c) Prolonged exposure to light. Explanation: Certain specimens, such as those for bilirubin tests, can be photosensitive. Prolonged exposure to light can degrade the specimen, compromising the accuracy of test results.

557. How can a phlebotomist ensure proper handling of specimens after collection?
a) By storing all specimens at room temperature
b) By delaying the labeling of specimens
c) By using appropriate storage conditions for different types of specimens
d) By transporting all specimens in the same container

Answer: c) By using appropriate storage conditions for different types of specimens. Explanation: Different types of specimens require different storage conditions. Following these requirements can help maintain specimen integrity.

558. Which of the following is NOT a proper step for preserving the integrity of collected specimens?
a) Transporting specimens to the lab as quickly as possible
b) Labeling specimens immediately after collection
c) Exposing light-sensitive specimens to light
d) Storing specimens at appropriate temperatures

Answer: c) Exposing light-sensitive specimens to light. Explanation: Light-sensitive specimens should be protected from light to maintain their integrity.

559. What is the primary reason for ensuring proper specimen handling in a clinical laboratory setting?
a) To make the job of a phlebotomist easier
b) To ensure the accuracy of test results
c) To reduce the need for specimen labeling
d) To decrease the time it takes to perform tests

Answer: b) To ensure the accuracy of test results. Explanation: Proper specimen handling is crucial to maintaining the integrity of the specimen and ensuring the accuracy of test results.

560. What is a potential consequence of mishandling specimens after collection?
a) Faster test results
b) Increased patient satisfaction
c) Misdiagnosis of a condition
d) Increased specimen quantity

Answer: c) Misdiagnosis of a condition. Explanation: Mishandling specimens can lead to inaccurate test results, which can in turn lead to misdiagnosis of a patient's condition.

561. Which of the following practices can affect the integrity of collected specimens?
a) Using clean and sterile equipment for collection
b) Transporting specimens to the lab immediately after collection
c) Storing specimens in a warm environment
d) Labeling specimens immediately after collection

Answer: c) Storing specimens in a warm environment. Explanation: Certain specimens require cool or even freezing temperatures for storage. Storing these specimens in a warm environment can compromise their integrity.

562. Why is it important to label specimens immediately after collection?
a) To ensure they are transported immediately
b) To prevent misidentification or mix-ups
c) To speed up the testing process
d) To increase the volume of the specimen

Answer: b) To prevent misidentification or mix-ups. Explanation: Proper labeling helps to ensure that each specimen can be correctly linked to the right patient, reducing the chances of errors or mix-ups.

563. What can happen if a blood sample for a glucose test is left at room temperature for an extended period of time?
a) The glucose levels in the sample may increase
b) The glucose levels in the sample will remain unchanged
c) The glucose levels in the sample may decrease
d) The glucose levels in the sample will fluctuate randomly

Answer: c) The glucose levels in the sample may decrease. Explanation: If a blood sample for a glucose test is left at room temperature for an extended period of time, the glucose in the sample can be consumed by cells, potentially leading to falsely low glucose measurements.

564. Which of the following is NOT a method to mitigate factors that can affect the integrity of specimens after collection?
a) Using specific preservatives for certain types of specimens
b) Storing all specimens at room temperature
c) Labeling specimens immediately after collection
d) Transporting specimens to the lab as soon as possible

Answer: b) Storing all specimens at room temperature. Explanation: Not all specimens should be stored at room temperature. Different types of specimens may require specific storage conditions to maintain their integrity.

565. What is a critical step to be taken immediately after the collection of blood specimens to ensure their integrity?
a) Labeling the specimens
b) Placing them in a cooler
c) Leaving them at room temperature
d) Shaking them vigorously

Answer: a) Labeling the specimens. Explanation: Specimens should be labeled immediately after collection, including patient identification information, date and time of collection, and the collector's initials. This ensures the specimens are correctly linked to the patient and helps prevent mix-ups or errors.

566. When packaging blood specimens for transport, what is an important factor to consider?
a) The size of the package
b) The specimen type and its storage requirements
c) The color of the packaging
d) The weight of the packaging

Answer: b) The specimen type and its storage requirements. Explanation: Different specimens have different storage requirements to maintain their integrity. It's crucial to package specimens in a way that meets these requirements, such as refrigeration or protection from light.

567. What information should be included when labeling a blood specimen?
a) Patient's full name, date, and time of collection
b) Patient's full name, medical history, and time of collection
c) Patient's full name, age, and blood type
d) Patient's full name, address, and date of collection

Answer: a) Patient's full name, date, and time of collection. Explanation: When labeling a blood specimen, it's critical to include the patient's full name, date, and time of collection. This helps ensure accurate patient identification and proper specimen handling.

568. What guidelines should be followed when transporting specimens within a healthcare facility?
a) The specimens should be transported by the fastest route possible, even if it means running through crowded areas
b) The specimens should be transported without any packaging
c) The specimens should be transported in a sturdy, leak-proof container and in a manner that maintains their appropriate temperature
d) The specimens should be transported by the patient themselves

Answer: c) The specimens should be transported in a sturdy, leak-proof container and in a manner that maintains their appropriate temperature. Explanation: For internal transport, specimens should be securely packaged in leak-proof containers, and the necessary temperature conditions should be maintained.

569. How does transporting specimens to an external lab differ from transporting specimens within a facility?
a) No difference; the same procedures apply
b) External transport requires additional documentation and may need specialized packaging for maintaining temperature conditions
c) External transport is faster than internal transport
d) External transport does not require any packaging

Answer: b) External transport requires additional documentation and may need specialized packaging for maintaining temperature conditions. Explanation: When transporting specimens to an external lab, there may be additional requirements for documentation, as well as more specific needs for packaging and temperature control.

570. What is the primary goal of proper specimen handling and transportation procedures?
a) To make the process faster
b) To ensure the accuracy of test results
c) To reduce the workload of the laboratory staff
d) To save costs on specimen storage

Answer: b) To ensure the accuracy of test results. Explanation: Proper handling and transport of specimens are vital to maintain their integrity and ensure the accuracy of test results.

571. What potential issue can arise from improper labeling of blood specimens?
a) It can lead to a delay in transportation
b) It can lead to the loss of the specimen
c) It can lead to errors in patient identification and incorrect test results
d) It can lead to a quicker testing process

Answer: c) It can lead to errors in patient identification and incorrect test results. Explanation: Improper labeling can result in the specimen being linked to the wrong patient, which could lead to incorrect test results and potentially incorrect treatment.

572. How should a phlebotomist handle a blood specimen that needs to be refrigerated if immediate refrigeration is not possible?
a) The specimen should be placed in a cooler with ice packs
b) The specimen should be kept at room temperature
c) The specimen should be frozen
d) The specimen should be discarded

Answer: a) The specimen should be placed in a cooler with ice packs. Explanation: If immediate refrigeration is not available, a cooler with ice packs can be used to maintain the appropriate temperature for the specimen.

573. When packaging specimens for transport, why is it important to use a leak-proof container?
a) To prevent contamination of other specimens
b) To comply with regulations
c) To prevent loss of the specimen and protect transport personnel from potential exposure to the specimen
d) All of the above

Answer: d) All of the above. Explanation: Using a leak-proof container prevents the specimen from contaminating other specimens or the transport environment, complies with safety and health regulations, and protects the people handling the specimen from potential exposure.

574. What is one of the risks associated with not maintaining the appropriate temperature for a specimen during transport?
a) It can lead to an increase in the specimen's volume
b) It can lead to changes in the specimen that may affect test results
c) It can cause the specimen to change color
d) It can cause the specimen to become less infectious

Answer: b) It can lead to changes in the specimen that may affect test results. Explanation: If a specimen is not kept at the appropriate temperature, it may undergo changes that could affect the accuracy of test results.

575. When storing blood specimens, which factor is important to consider?
a) The time of collection
b) The type of test to be performed
c) The color of the specimen tube
d) The size of the specimen tube

Answer: b) The type of test to be performed. Explanation: The type of test to be performed on the specimen often determines the storage conditions required to maintain its integrity, such as temperature and light exposure.

576. Which type of test typically requires the specimen to be frozen for storage?
a) Complete blood count (CBC)
b) Glucose testing
c) Hormone testing
d) Coagulation testing

Answer: c) Hormone testing. Explanation: Many hormone tests require the specimen to be frozen to preserve the stability of the hormones. Other tests, such as CBC, glucose, and coagulation tests, typically do not require freezing.

577. What is the recommended temperature for refrigerating blood specimens?
a) Below freezing
b) 2-8 degrees Celsius (35.6-46.4 degrees Fahrenheit)
c) Room temperature
d) 10-15 degrees Celsius (50-59 degrees Fahrenheit)

Answer: b) 2-8 degrees Celsius (35.6-46.4 degrees Fahrenheit). Explanation: The recommended temperature for refrigerating blood specimens is typically 2-8 degrees Celsius. This helps preserve the integrity of the specimen for specific tests.

578. When is it appropriate to store a blood specimen at room temperature?
a) When the specimen is for a glucose test
b) When the specimen is for a coagulation test
c) When the specimen is for a complete blood count (CBC)
d) When the specimen is for a hormone test

Answer: c) When the specimen is for a complete blood count (CBC). Explanation: Blood specimens for a CBC are typically stored at room temperature.

579. What is a common mistake to avoid when storing blood specimens in the refrigerator?
a) Storing them in the door of the refrigerator
b) Storing them in airtight containers
c) Storing them at the back of the refrigerator
d) Storing them in the middle of the refrigerator

Answer: a) Storing them in the door of the refrigerator. Explanation: Storing specimens in the door of the refrigerator should be avoided because the temperature there can fluctuate more than in other parts of the refrigerator.

580. What could be the consequence of not properly thawing a frozen blood specimen before testing?
a) The specimen will be too cold to handle
b) The specimen will be diluted
c) The test results could be inaccurate
d) The specimen will become contaminated

Answer: c) The test results could be inaccurate. Explanation: If a frozen specimen is not properly thawed before testing, it may impact the test results, leading to inaccurate results.

581. How can phlebotomists avoid confusion when storing multiple specimens in the same refrigerator?
a) By writing their names on the specimens
b) By using color-coded containers
c) By storing all specimens together
d) By organizing specimens by patient and test type

Answer: d) By organizing specimens by patient and test type. Explanation: Organizing specimens by patient and test type can help reduce confusion and mix-ups, which in turn helps ensure the accuracy of test results.

582. What is a potential risk of storing a blood specimen at an incorrect temperature?
a) The specimen may change color
b) The specimen may lose volume
c) The specimen may alter in a way that affects the accuracy of test results
d) The specimen may become more infectious

Answer: c) The specimen may alter in a way that affects the accuracy of test results. Explanation: Storing a specimen at the wrong temperature could cause changes in the specimen that may impact the accuracy of test results.

583. What is an important factor to remember when storing a specimen for microbiological testing?
a) The specimen should be stored at room temperature
b) The specimen should be stored in a light-proof container
c) The specimen should be stored as quickly as possible
d) The specimen should be frozen

Answer: c) The specimen should be stored as quickly as possible. Explanation: Microbiological specimens are often sensitive to time and should be processed and stored as quickly as possible to prevent the growth or death of microorganisms.

584. Which of the following is not a recommended practice for handling specimens that need to be refrigerated or frozen?
a) Refrigerate or freeze the specimen as soon as possible after collection
b) Ensure the refrigerator or freezer is set to the correct temperature
c) Use a leak-proof container
d) Let the specimen sit at room temperature for a while before refrigeration or freezing

Answer: d) Let the specimen sit at room temperature for a while before refrigeration or freezing. Explanation: Specimens that need to be refrigerated or frozen should be placed in the refrigerator or freezer as soon as possible after collection. Letting them sit at room temperature could affect the specimen's integrity and the accuracy of test results.

585. In the context of specimen handling, what does 'chain of custody' refer to?
a) The order in which specimens are tested
b) The sequence of people who have handled a specimen
c) The tracking of a specimen's location over time
d) The prioritization of different specimens

Answer: b) The sequence of people who have handled a specimen. Explanation: 'Chain of custody' refers to the process of keeping up-to-date records of who has handled a specimen from the time it is collected to the time it is disposed of. This is crucial in cases like drug testing or forensic samples, where it is important to be able to prove that the specimen has not been tampered with.

586. Why is maintaining a chain of custody important in drug testing or forensic samples?
a) To ensure the accuracy of test results
b) To prevent contamination of the specimen
c) To protect patient confidentiality
d) To verify the identity of the person tested

Answer: d) To verify the identity of the person tested. Explanation: The chain of custody ensures that the specimen tested is indeed from the intended individual and that it has not been tampered with or contaminated. This is critical in situations like drug testing and forensic investigations.

587. What should be done immediately following a spill or breakage of specimens during transportation?
a) Leave the area immediately
b) Notify the laboratory supervisor
c) Collect the broken pieces
d) Try to recover the spilled specimen

Answer: b) Notify the laboratory supervisor. Explanation: In the event of a spill or breakage, the first step is to notify the appropriate supervisor or safety officer. They will provide guidance on the next steps based on the nature of the specimen and the spill.

588. What safety measure should be taken when handling broken specimen containers?
a) Wear gloves and use a tool to pick up broken pieces
b) Use bare hands to carefully collect the broken pieces
c) Sweep the broken pieces into a dustpan
d) Leave the broken pieces for someone else to clean up

Answer: a) Wear gloves and use a tool to pick up broken pieces. Explanation: Personal protective equipment, such as gloves, should be worn when handling broken specimen containers to prevent injury and exposure to potentially hazardous materials.

589. What should be used to clean up a spill of biological specimens?
a) Water
b) Bleach solution
c) Alcohol wipes
d) Window cleaner

Answer: b) Bleach solution. Explanation: A bleach solution is typically recommended for cleaning up spills of biological specimens because it can kill a wide variety of microorganisms.

590. What is the most important thing to do after a specimen spill has been cleaned up?
a) Wash your hands
b) Dispose of the cleanup materials properly
c) Document the incident
d) Notify the patient

Answer: c) Document the incident. Explanation: While all the options are important, documenting the incident is crucial. This documentation can help identify patterns or areas for improvement in specimen handling and transportation.

591. Why is it important to wear personal protective equipment (PPE) when transporting specimens?
a) To keep the specimens clean
b) To protect oneself from potential exposure to harmful substances
c) To appear professional
d) To maintain the chain of custody

Answer: b) To protect oneself from potential exposure to harmful substances. Explanation: Wearing PPE, such as gloves and lab coats, can protect against exposure to potentially harmful substances in the specimens being transported.

592. In the context of specimen handling, which of the following scenarios requires the implementation of a chain of custody?
a) A blood sample collected for a routine complete blood count (CBC)
b) A urine sample collected for a routine urinalysis
c) A blood sample collected for a routine blood chemistry panel
d) A urine sample collected for a drug test

Answer: d) A urine sample collected for a drug test. Explanation: Chain of custody is usually required for legal or forensic cases, such as drug tests, where it is crucial to verify that the specimen was indeed collected from the person identified and that it hasn't been tampered with.

593. What is the best way to maintain the chain of custody of a specimen?
a) Collecting the specimen in the presence of a witness
b) Having each person who handles the specimen sign a log
c) Keeping the specimen in a locked container at all times
d) Taking a photo of the person from whom the specimen was collected

Answer: b) Having each person who handles the specimen sign a log. Explanation: The chain of custody is maintained by documenting each person who has handled the specimen. This is typically done through a log or form that is signed by each individual who takes custody of the specimen.

594. In the context of a clinical laboratory, what does specimen processing primarily entail?
a) Collection of specimens from patients
b) Transport of specimens to the laboratory
c) Preparation of specimens for analysis
d) Interpretation of test results

Answer: c) Preparation of specimens for analysis. Explanation: Specimen processing refers to the steps taken after specimen collection and before testing to prepare specimens for analysis. This may include labeling, sorting, centrifuging, aliquoting, and storing specimens.

595. What is a common first step in specimen processing in the laboratory?
a) Performing the test immediately
b) Centrifuging the specimen
c) Recording the specimen's arrival in the laboratory information system
d) Refrigerating the specimen

Answer: c) Recording the specimen's arrival in the laboratory information system. Explanation: The first step in specimen processing is typically recording the arrival of the specimen in the lab, including the time of arrival and the condition of the specimen. This provides a record of when the specimen was received and can help ensure the timely processing of the specimen.

596. What is the primary purpose of centrifuging a blood specimen during processing?
a) To mix the blood with the anticoagulant in the tube
b) To separate the blood cells from the serum or plasma
c) To kill any bacteria present in the blood
d) To speed up the clotting process

Answer: b) To separate the blood cells from the serum or plasma. Explanation: Centrifuging a blood specimen spins it at a high speed, causing the heavier blood cells to settle at the bottom of the tube and the lighter serum or plasma to rise to the top. This separation allows for the testing of the serum or plasma without interference from the cells.

597. How does the processing of a urine specimen typically differ from that of a blood specimen?
a) Urine specimens need to be centrifuged, but blood specimens do not
b) Urine specimens must be kept at body temperature, while blood specimens can be stored at room temperature
c) Urine specimens are often tested immediately, while blood specimens may be stored for later testing
d) Urine specimens require a different type of collection container than blood specimens

Answer: c) Urine specimens are often tested immediately, while blood specimens may be stored for later testing. Explanation: While both types of specimens may need to be processed before testing, urine tests are often performed immediately after collection, while blood tests may be performed later.

598. Why are tissue specimens often fixed in formalin during processing?
a) To sterilize the tissue
b) To enhance the color of the tissue
c) To preserve the tissue's structure
d) To dissolve any fat in the tissue

Answer: c) To preserve the tissue's structure. Explanation: Fixing a tissue specimen in formalin helps preserve the tissue's structure and prevents decay. This is crucial for histology, where the microscopic structure of the tissue is being examined.

599. Which type of specimen would most likely require embedding in paraffin wax during processing?
a) Blood
b) Urine
c) Saliva
d) Tissue

Answer: d) Tissue. Explanation: Tissue specimens are often embedded in paraffin wax during processing. This provides support and enables thin sections to be cut for microscopic examination.

600. What is a primary reason for staining tissue specimens during processing?
a) To make the specimens more visually appealing
b) To kill any bacteria present in the specimens
c) To enhance contrast and highlight different structures under the microscope
d) To speed up the processing time

Answer: c) To enhance contrast and highlight different structures under the microscope. Explanation: Staining is used in histology to differentiate various elements of the tissue. Different stains bind to different types of tissues and cells, making them easier to distinguish under a microscope.

601. Which of the following is an important consideration when aliquoting a specimen for multiple tests?
a) The patient's age and sex
b) The time the specimen was collected
c) The volume of specimen required for each test
d) The color of the specimen

Answer: c) The volume of specimen required for each test. Explanation: It's essential to know how much of the specimen each test requires to ensure there is enough specimen for all tests. If there is not enough, the tests may need to be prioritized or more specimen collected.

602. What is a common step in processing a blood culture specimen?
a) Embedding the blood in paraffin wax
b) Incubating the blood at body temperature
c) Staining the blood with a special dye
d) Centrifuging the blood to separate the cells

Answer: b) Incubating the blood at body temperature. Explanation: Blood culture specimens are typically incubated at body temperature to encourage the growth of any bacteria present in the blood. This allows for the detection of bacteria that are causing an infection in the patient's bloodstream.

603. What is the primary purpose of centrifugation in specimen processing?
a) To mix the sample thoroughly
b) To cool the sample before testing
c) To separate components based on density
d) To sterilize the sample before testing

Answer: c) To separate components based on density. Explanation: Centrifugation spins the sample at high speeds, causing the components of different densities to separate. This is crucial in many tests, such as those that require serum or plasma, which can be isolated from whole blood through centrifugation.

604. What precaution should be taken when centrifuging a specimen?
a) The centrifuge should be balanced
b) The centrifuge should be sterilized between each use
c) The centrifuge should be cooled to a specific temperature
d) The centrifuge should be calibrated after each use

Answer: a) The centrifuge should be balanced. Explanation: When using a centrifuge, it is crucial to balance the load to prevent damage to the centrifuge and to ensure accurate results. This is usually done by placing tubes of equal weight opposite each other in the centrifuge rotor.

605. What does aliquoting refer to in specimen processing?
a) Staining of a sample for microscopic examination
b) Division of a sample into smaller portions for testing
c) Heating of a sample to a specific temperature
d) Addition of a reagent to a sample

Answer: b) Division of a sample into smaller portions for testing. Explanation: Aliquoting involves dividing a sample into smaller portions, each of which can be used for a separate test. This is often necessary when multiple tests need to be performed on a single sample.

606. What is the correct technique for aliquoting a sample?
a) Pouring the sample into test tubes
b) Using a pipette to transfer the sample
c) Dipping a swab into the sample
d) Scooping the sample with a spatula

Answer: b) Using a pipette to transfer the sample. Explanation: The correct technique for aliquoting a sample typically involves using a pipette to accurately measure and transfer the desired amount of sample into a new container. This helps to prevent contamination and ensures that the correct volume of sample is used for each test.

607. What information typically needs to be entered into the laboratory information system during specimen processing?
a) The patient's medical history
b) The test results
c) The time and date of specimen arrival
d) The patient's insurance information

Answer: c) The time and date of specimen arrival. Explanation: When a specimen arrives in the laboratory, the time and date of arrival are typically entered into the laboratory information system. This helps to track the specimen and ensures that it is processed in a timely manner.

608. Which of the following is a common error to avoid when entering data into the laboratory information system?
a) Entering data too quickly
b) Using medical abbreviations
c) Double-checking all entries
d) Entering data in the wrong patient's record

Answer: d) Entering data in the wrong patient's record. Explanation: It's crucial to ensure that data is entered in the correct patient's record. Errors can result in misdiagnosis, inappropriate treatment, or other serious consequences.

609. Why is it important to record the condition of the specimen upon arrival in the laboratory?
a) To determine the patient's diagnosis
b) To know how to process the specimen
c) To identify any potential pre-analytical errors
d) To confirm the patient's identity

Answer: c) To identify any potential pre-analytical errors. Explanation: Recording the condition of the specimen upon arrival can help identify any pre-analytical errors such as hemolysis or clotting in a blood sample. These errors can affect the test results and need to be noted.

610. When aliquoting, why should you avoid touching the pipette tip to the sides of the tube or container?
a) It can cause the sample to clot
b) It can lead to contamination of the sample
c) It can alter the test results
d) It can cause the sample to evaporate

Answer: b) It can lead to contamination of the sample. Explanation: Touching the pipette tip to the sides of the tube or container can lead to contamination of the sample, which could affect the test results.

611. Why is it important to centrifuge a specimen promptly after collection?
a) To prevent the sample from clotting
b) To kill any bacteria in the sample
c) To enhance the sample's color
d) To prevent the breakdown of cells and analytes

Answer: d) To prevent the breakdown of cells and analytes. Explanation: If a specimen is not centrifuged promptly after collection, cells and analytes may start to break down, which could affect the test results. Centrifuging the specimen promptly helps to separate the cells from the plasma or serum, preserving the integrity of the specimen.

612. Which of the following would not be a standard step in the data entry process during specimen processing?
a) Recording the patient's name and date of birth
b) Documenting the color and consistency of the specimen
c) Inputting the tests to be performed on the specimen
d) Writing a preliminary diagnosis based on the appearance of the specimen

Answer: d) Writing a preliminary diagnosis based on the appearance of the specimen. Explanation: The data entry process typically involves recording identifying information about the patient and the specimen, as well as the tests to be performed. A preliminary diagnosis would not usually be made at this stage, as this requires analysis of the specimen and interpretation of the test results.

613. A common error in specimen processing that can compromise test results is:
a) Not labeling the specimen immediately after collection
b) Not storing the specimen at the right temperature
c) Not taking the patient's medical history before collection
d) Not sterilizing the collection site adequately

Answer: b) Not storing the specimen at the right temperature. Explanation: Proper storage conditions are vital to maintain the integrity of a specimen. Incorrect temperature can cause changes in the specimen that may affect the test results.

614. Which of the following is an effective way for phlebotomists to prevent errors during specimen processing?
a) Perform all tests as soon as the specimen is collected
b) Use only automated equipment to avoid human error
c) Double-check patient and specimen information
d) Skip unnecessary quality control procedures to save time

Answer: c) Double-check patient and specimen information. Explanation: One of the key responsibilities of a phlebotomist is to ensure that the patient and specimen information is accurate. This includes the patient's identity, the type and condition of the specimen, and the tests ordered.

615. A critical quality control measure in the specimen processing area is:
a) Having a designated area for food and drink
b) Regular inspection and maintenance of equipment
c) Having a comfortable chair for the phlebotomist
d) Keeping the windows open for ventilation

Answer: b) Regular inspection and maintenance of equipment. Explanation: Regular maintenance and inspection of the equipment ensure that they function correctly and give reliable results. Any equipment malfunction can compromise the quality of the test results.

616. Maintaining and cleaning equipment used in specimen processing contributes to laboratory safety by:
a) Making the equipment look clean and professional
b) Ensuring that the equipment functions properly
c) Keeping the laboratory smelling fresh
d) Making the equipment lighter and easier to move

Answer: b) Ensuring that the equipment functions properly. Explanation: Regular cleaning and maintenance can prevent equipment malfunction, which could cause accidents or compromise safety. It also prevents cross-contamination, ensuring accurate and reliable test results.

617. Which of the following is NOT a common error during specimen processing?
a) Mislabeling of specimens
b) Inappropriate specimen storage
c) Not following aseptic techniques
d) Keeping a detailed patient diary

Answer: d) Keeping a detailed patient diary. Explanation: Phlebotomists and laboratory staff do not typically keep a detailed patient diary. Instead, they focus on accurately documenting specimen-related information.

618. Quality assurance in the specimen processing area can be improved by:
a) Running control samples alongside patient specimens
b) Performing all tests manually
c) Using the same reagents for all tests
d) Ignoring minor equipment malfunctions

Answer: a) Running control samples alongside patient specimens. Explanation: Control samples have known values and serve as a gauge to determine if the test is working properly. If the control sample result is within the expected range, it confirms that the testing process is accurate and reliable.

619. Routine cleaning of specimen processing equipment contributes to quality assurance by:
a) Increasing the lifespan of the equipment
b) Ensuring accurate and reliable test results
c) Making the laboratory look neat and organized
d) Keeping the laboratory well-stocked with cleaning supplies

Answer: b) Ensuring accurate and reliable test results. Explanation: Regular cleaning of equipment prevents the buildup of residue or contaminants that could interfere with the test results, ensuring that they are accurate and reliable.

620. A common way for phlebotomists to prevent errors in specimen processing is:
a) Running all tests twice
b) Mixing up samples to test their adaptability
c) Verifying patient and test information
d) Storing all samples at room temperature

Answer: c) Verifying patient and test information.

621. When a phlebotomist fails to adequately mix an anticoagulant tube after drawing a blood sample, this may lead to:
a) Hemolysis
b) Lipemia
c) Clotting
d) Icterus

Answer: c) Clotting. Explanation: Inadequate mixing can prevent the anticoagulant from fully interacting with the blood, which can then lead to clotting.

622. A potential error that could occur during specimen processing is:
a) Using a new needle for every patient
b) Verifying the patient's identification before collection
c) Mishandling or mislabeling of the specimen
d) Cleaning the venipuncture site before collection

Answer: c) Mishandling or mislabeling of the specimen. Explanation: Mishandling or mislabeling of specimens could lead to errors in patient identification, which may result in incorrect test results or treatments.

623. Which of the following is an essential quality control measure in specimen processing?
a) Testing samples immediately after collection
b) Using the same batch of reagents for all tests
c) Implementing a system of double checks for labeling
d) Refrigerating all samples, regardless of the recommended storage conditions

Answer: c) Implementing a system of double checks for labeling. Explanation: Mistakes in labeling can lead to serious errors, so having a system of double checks ensures that the correct patient's sample is being processed and tested.

624. A critical aspect of maintaining equipment used in specimen processing is:
a) Applying a fresh coat of paint regularly
b) Cleaning and sanitizing surfaces after each use
c) Ensuring the equipment is aesthetically pleasing
d) Replacing equipment every year, regardless of condition

Answer: b) Cleaning and sanitizing surfaces after each use. Explanation: Regular cleaning prevents contamination, ensuring the accuracy of results and reducing the spread of infection.

625. To ensure the reliability and accuracy of test results, the laboratory should:
a) Use a single supplier for all its reagents
b) Employ the same team of staff for all tests
c) Implement regular calibration and maintenance of equipment
d) Only accept specimens collected by experienced phlebotomists

Answer: c) Implement regular calibration and maintenance of equipment. Explanation: Regular calibration and maintenance ensure that equipment is functioning correctly, which is crucial for reliable and accurate test results.

626. Which of the following could significantly affect the integrity of a blood sample during processing?
a) Applying a bandage to the venipuncture site
b) Storing the sample at an incorrect temperature
c) Verifying the patient's identity before collection
d) Using a needle of appropriate size for the venipuncture

Answer: b) Storing the sample at an incorrect temperature. Explanation: The temperature at which a specimen is stored can greatly impact the stability of certain components, affecting the accuracy of test results.

627. A significant part of quality assurance in the laboratory involves:
a) Testing as many samples as possible within a given timeframe
b) Relying solely on automated machines to avoid human error
c) Strict adherence to established protocols and procedures
d) Keeping the work environment as quiet as possible to avoid distractions

Answer: c) Strict adherence to established protocols and procedures. Explanation: Following established protocols ensures consistency and accuracy in test results, contributing to high-quality patient care.

628. One way to prevent errors in specimen processing is by:
a) Running tests even when control samples have not yielded expected results
b) Strictly adhering to a first-in, first-out system for processing samples
c) Only accepting samples from patients who are well-hydrated
d) Completing paperwork for samples before they are collected

Answer: b) Strictly adhering to a first-in, first-out system for processing samples

629. Rachel, a phlebotomist, has just finished collecting blood samples from a patient who is suspected of having a bacterial infection. What should be Rachel's next step in handling the blood culture bottles?
a) Leaving them at room temperature for 30 minutes before processing.
b) Immediately incubating the bottles to promote bacterial growth.
c) Storing the bottles in a refrigerator until ready for testing.
d) Shaking the bottles vigorously to mix the contents.

Answer: b) Immediately incubating the bottles to promote bacterial growth. Explanation: Blood culture bottles are incubated to promote the growth of bacteria, which is essential for identifying bacterial infections. Immediate incubation ensures optimal conditions for bacterial growth.

630. Jack, a laboratory technician, receives a blood specimen to be tested for glucose levels but notices that the sample is hemolyzed. What should he do?
a) Proceed with the glucose test, assuming the hemolysis won't affect the results.
b) Discard the sample and ask the phlebotomist to collect a new one.
c) Centrifuge the sample and use the plasma for testing.
d) Refrigerate the sample and test it later when there's less workload.

Answer: b) Discard the sample and ask the phlebotomist to collect a new one. Explanation: Hemolysis can affect the accuracy of many laboratory tests, including glucose. A new sample should be collected to ensure accurate test results.

631. Hannah, a phlebotomist, is tasked with processing a urine sample for a drug screen. The specimen must maintain a chain of custody. What should Hannah do to ensure this?
a) Label the specimen with the patient's name and date of collection.
b) Document every person who handles the specimen and ensure it's sealed properly.
c) Centrifuge the urine specimen before storing it.
d) Ensure the specimen is stored at room temperature.

Answer: b) Document every person who handles the specimen and ensure it's sealed properly.
Explanation: Chain of custody requires documentation of every person who handles the specimen and proper sealing to ensure that there has been no tampering.

632. Andrew, a phlebotomist, accidentally spills a blood specimen on the floor of the lab. What is the first step he should take in response to this incident?
a) Use paper towels to clean up the spill.
b) Notify his supervisor about the incident.
c) Put on gloves and use a disinfectant to clean up the spill.
d) Leave the area immediately and let someone else handle it.

Answer: c) Put on gloves and use a disinfectant to clean up the spill. Explanation: It is crucial to prioritize safety by using personal protective equipment and properly disinfecting the area to minimize the risk of exposure to bloodborne pathogens.

633. Linda, a lab technician, notices that the centrifuge used for processing blood samples is making an unusual noise. What should be her immediate course of action?
a) Continue to use the centrifuge but wear earplugs to block the noise.
b) Report the issue to a supervisor and discontinue use until it is inspected.
c) Try to fix the centrifuge herself.
d) Ignore the noise and assume it's normal for the centrifuge.

Answer: b) Report the issue to a supervisor and discontinue use until it is inspected. Explanation: The unusual noise might indicate a malfunction. Using a malfunctioning centrifuge can lead to erroneous results or pose a safety hazard.

634. Catherine, a lab technician, has been asked to aliquot a plasma sample into multiple tubes for various tests. What should Catherine ensure before aliquoting the sample?
a) The primary specimen tube is properly mixed.
b) She is using the largest pipette available.
c) All aliquot tubes are pre-labeled with the patient's name.
d) She freezes the original sample before aliquoting.

Answer: a) The primary specimen tube is properly mixed. Explanation: Proper mixing ensures a homogeneous sample, which is crucial for accurate test results when aliquoting.

635. A clinical laboratory received a blood sample with an unknown source of error. What quality control measure could potentially identify the source of the error?
a) Testing the sample immediately.
b) Verifying the patient's identity.
c) Repeating the test using a control sample.
d) Storing the sample at room temperature.

Answer: c) Repeating the test using a control sample. Explanation: Control samples, which have known values, can help identify if an error exists in the testing procedure, and could therefore potentially identify the source of the error in the patient's sample.

636. Emma, a phlebotomist, realizes she forgot to write the time of collection on a blood sample for a peak therapeutic drug level. What should Emma do?
a) Estimate the time of collection and write it on the label.
b) Leave it blank as it is not that important.
c) Notify the lab and collect a new sample if possible.
d) Write the current time on the label.

Answer: c) Notify the lab and collect a new sample if possible. Explanation: The collection time is crucial for therapeutic drug level testing as it's related to the drug's pharmacokinetics. If the correct time is not known, a new sample should be collected if possible.

637. Amanda, a lab technician, is tasked with cleaning and maintaining the equipment used in specimen processing. What should be included in Amanda's routine?
a) Regular cleaning, disinfection, and scheduled maintenance.
b) Replacing all equipment yearly.
c) Daily lubrication of all moving parts.
d) Use of household cleaners for routine cleaning.

Answer: a) Regular cleaning, disinfection, and scheduled maintenance. Explanation: Regular cleaning, disinfection, and scheduled maintenance are necessary to ensure the equipment functions correctly, and results from this equipment are accurate.

Embarking on this enlightening journey through the world of phlebotomy, you have demonstrated an admirable dedication to mastering a noble profession. The twists and turns of this path might have seemed daunting at first, but your perseverance, fueled by your aspiration, has carried you through. So, let's take a moment to reflect on the milestones we have crossed together.

From the meticulous steps involved in preparing for a venipuncture, navigating patient interactions, adhering to stringent infection control measures, to understanding the complexity of blood and its components, we've covered a vast terrain. And we didn't stop there. We delved deeper into therapeutic phlebotomy, honing your expertise in POCT, and immersed ourselves in the nitty-gritty of specimen processing and handling. These insights will be your lighthouse in the tempestuous sea of professional challenges.

It's natural to falter, to feel the sting of error, but remember, each stumble is not a failure, but a lesson engraved in the slate of your experience. Embrace them not as setbacks, but as stepping stones, sculpting your path towards excellence.

As the exam draws near, it's alright to sense a flutter of anxiety, an echo of doubt. It's a testament to your care for the work you aspire to do. Channel this energy into your final preparations, allow it to sharpen your focus, and remember, fear is a mountain best conquered by steadily climbing one step at a time.

Remember those moments when a pattern emerged, a piece of knowledge suddenly clicked into place, and your suspicions transformed into understanding? Hold onto those moments, they are the sparks that will ignite your intuitive skill, allowing you to connect the dots in real-life scenarios.

The realm of phlebotomy is not without its adversaries - unforeseen complications, challenging patients, and demanding situations. Together, we've explored strategies to turn these adversaries into opportunities, arming you with the right knowledge stones to throw in the face of these challenges.

As we close this chapter of your study journey, know that you are not alone. We stand with you, applauding your efforts, celebrating your determination, and eagerly anticipating your success. When you step into that exam room, remember that you're not merely proving your skills and knowledge, you're showcasing the tireless commitment that brought you this far.

My heartfelt wishes accompany you as you cross this pivotal threshold. May your endeavors be fruitful, and may the triumph be as gratifying as the journey itself. Be proud, be confident, and seize the day!

216

9 781088 198810